Also by Dawn Freshwater:

Counselling Skills for Nurses, Midwives and Health Visitors (2003)
Emotions and Needs (2002) with C. Robertson
*Therapeutic Nursing: Improving Patient Care Through
   Self-awareness and Reflection* (2002)
*Critical Reflection for Nursing and the Helping Professions:
   A User's Guide* (2001) with G. Rolfe and M. Jasper*
Transforming Nursing Through Reflective Practice (1998)
   with C. Johns

Also by Veronica Bishop:

*Challenges in Clinical Practice: Professional Developments
   in Nursing* (2000) with I. Scott*
*Clinical Supervision in Practice: Some Questions, Answers
   and Guidelines* (1998)*

* Also published by Palgrave Macmillan

Nursing Research in Context

Appreciation, Application and Professional Development

Edited by

Dawn Freshwater

and

Veronica Bishop

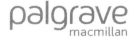

First published 2004 by
PALGRAVE MACMILLAN
Houndmills, Basingstoke, Hampshire RG21 6XS and
175 Fifth Avenue, New York, N.Y. 10010
Companies and representatives throughout the world

PALGRAVE MACMILLAN is the global academic imprint of the
Palgrave Macmillan division of St. Martin's Press LLC and of Palgrave
Macmillan Ltd. Macmillan® is a registered trademark in the United
States, United Kingdom and other countries. Palgrave is a registered
trademark in the European Union and other countries.

ISBN 0–333–99354–3 paperback

This book is printed on paper suitable for recycling and made from
fully managed and sustained forest sources.

A catalogue record for this book is available from the British Library.

10   9   8   7   6   5   4   3   2   1
12 11 10 09 08 07 06 05 04 13

Typeset in Great Britain by
Aarontype Ltd, Easton, Bristol

Printed and bound in Great Britain by
J.W. Arrowsmith Ltd, Bristol

Contents

Preface

The aim of this book is to provide a position paper on the state of nursing research in the early twenty-first century. We envisage that it will be of interest to students of policy as well as those concerned with the development of nursing research in general and with their personal professional development in particular. The book is pertinent to the novice and to the more experienced researcher as well as to those who seek to provide support systems between academia and service provision. It is divided into two parts – the first studies, in depth, the policy and professional issues impacting on research into nursing; the second takes the reader through the processes of professional development and career options. While dipping into a chapter on a 'needs must' basis will provide invaluable insights and advice, read as a whole the fascinating ribbon of professional progress is spread before the reader, from the inspirational to the specific.

The first chapter in Part I introduces the reader to the context of nursing research in the United Kingdom and, importantly, to current policy initiatives which impact on the profession. The rationale for nursing to develop a genuine culture of research that can enable the profession to deliver research-oriented practice is argued both from the ideology of professional working and from the need to clarify the nursing contribution to health care in a multidisciplinary environment. Links between research and clinical governance are made, and the text seeks to outline the wider implications for the position of nursing within the academy, within health care and in society.

Chapter 2 takes the discussion to a greater depth, discussing policy initiatives in the United Kingdom and the drive for capacity building in research and development in nursing and midwifery. Drawing on their study of key policy documents and processes the authors argue for a many-pronged approach to establish high-calibre research in these professions. The case is made that researchers, educators, managers and clinicians need to join forces with patient and user groups and that any investment in nursing and midwifery R&D will have failed if it only ever benefits the professional community.

Shifting the focus away from purely UK initiatives in nursing research, Chapter 3 widens the reader's perspective, highlighting that the organisation of nursing and health care within the UK is heavily influenced by a number of international agendas and agreements, often in negotiation with the World Health Organization (WHO) and members of the European community. The authors, who come from opposite sides of the Atlantic, explore some of the global networks that are available to nurses and consider the rewards of international professional/research collaboration. They stress that, now more than ever in the light of people moving across national boundaries with relative ease, shared knowledge is central to professional growth and progress in health care delivery. In whichever part of the world the reader may find him- or herself there are essential skills required in order to provide knowledgeable care. These include the ability to critique published or spoken works, and accessing and understanding the researcher's role; issues which are addressed in depth in Chapter 4. This chapter studies the processes of appreciation and evaluation, and explains commonly used terms such as clinical effectiveness and evidence-based care. The text is aimed at the novice as well as the more experienced researcher, discussing the essentials to the research processes. Chapter 5, the final chapter in Part I, leads from appreciation of research to the actual doing of it. In this sense Chapter 5 focuses on the pragmatic, providing practical information and guidance for researchers at all levels: how to define the research question?; which methodology to use? There is particular emphasis on the dynamics of carrying out research, and the desirability of good support mechanisms is stressed.

Part II begins with Chapter 6, which contends that, at its best, a doctoral programme involves discovering and disseminating knowledge to benefit practice and notes that in countries where nurses have been delayed in gaining admission to doctoral programmes the development of nursing knowledge has also been delayed. This chapter presents data on the processes of doctoral study, providing invaluable information about the various options now available, commenting on the processes and procedures as they are developing in nursing. Chapter 7 uniquely profiles five research-active nurses. These profiles are of particular relevance to the reader who is considering what opportunities exist to break into research, offering insights into how one might build on existing models. Career possibilities are discussed for both the novice and the more advanced researcher.

Chapter 8 takes the reader through the processes of developing a research portfolio, whether as part of an organisation-wide strategy, or the beginnings of an area of interest to the individual. This is complemented in Chapter 9 by identification of the essential issue of how to obtain funding for research. The advice offered ranges from how to obtain small grants and scholarships for personal development to how to approach major funding bodies such as the Department of Health and the Medical Research Council to support mainstream research activities. Having completed the research, the importance, indeed the ethical requirement, of publishing it is discussed. Chapter 10 provides useful practical advice, both for the beginner and for the more experienced on how to get your research published, and the need to communicate effectively between academia and the service is stressed.

Finally, the two editors use Chapter 11 to look ahead. In doing this they consider where the nursing profession is now, what has made a difference, and where achievement has not matched expectations. Combining a blue skies approach with pragmatism they consider how the profession should be moving forwards, in terms of both academic and clinical excellence. What are the potential elephant traps? What supporting mechanisms and enhancers need to be in place to make the nursing contribution to health and health care the most effective and the most appropriate for every individual? How do they envisage health care provision in the ongoing century and care in the NHS in particular? Bevan's dream of the NHS may not have encompassed nursing *per se* – but we are clear that its future is dependent on our professional success, and this book considers the potential mapping of that promise.

V.B.
D.F.

Acknowledgements

Our thanks go to the many researchers, practitioners and educationalists who have been willing to enter into discussion about the process of creating this book. In addition to those who have made specific contributions to the chapters, we wish to acknowledge the support and advice of Jon Reed, Magenta Lampson and the reviewers. As always, our families deserve special thanks, for their patience and understanding during the difficult times.

Notes on contributors

Veronica Bishop PhD MPhil RGN FRSA

Veronica is Editor of *Nursing Times Research*, the first academic journal in the UK to use open critique, and is a board member of the Hong Kong nurses' journal. She recently retired as Professor of Nursing, De Montfort University but maintains her links with the NHS through consultancy work, particularly in relation to clinical supervision on which she is widely published. This interest developed from her role as the lead Nursing Officer in the Department of Health for Nursing Development Units, innovations in clinical practice and clinical supervision. She spearheaded the strategic document 'Vision for the Future' (DoH, 1993) on the nursing and midwifery contribution to health, and set up the first national nursing practice database. Veronica has worked as a consultant for the World Health Organisation in Denmark, India and Romania, and is on the scientific committee of the RCN Research Society and an executive member of the Florence Nightingale Foundation.

Steven Ersser PhD BSc (Hons) RGN CertHEd

Steven is Head of Nursing Development and leads the Skin Vulnerability Research Group in the School of Nursing & Midwifery at the University of Southampton. Prior to this he was Reader in Nursing at Oxford Brookes University. He trained at Guy's Hospital, London and then took posts in Oxford in medical and elderly care and later dermatology, working as senior nurse/clinical lecturer in the Department of Dermatology. He also worked in the Oxford Nursing Development Unit and the National Institute for Nursing, integrating practice with research. His PhD, from King's College, University of London, focuses on nursing as a therapeutic activity. He has been a Visiting Scholar at St. John's College, Cambridge, and remains an Honorary Research Associate at the University of Sydney. Steven is the University's nursing link for R&D to the Southampton University

Hospitals Trust and is Research & International Advisor to the British Dermatological Nursing Group. He is co-founder and Chair of the International Skin Care Nursing Advisory Group, which is working on a project with World Health Organisation.

Dawn Freshwater PhD BA (Hons) RGN RNT FRCN

Dawn is Professor of Mental Health and Primary Care at IHCS Bournemouth University and is leading the development of an Academic Research Centre in Practice with North and South West Dorset NHS Trusts. Having completed her nurse training in 1983 she worked in both acute and community settings before undertaking her first degree at the Institute of Advanced Nurse Education, Royal College of Nursing, later completing her PhD at the University of Nottingham. The focus of her work has been on critical reflexivity, practice-based research and therapeutic practice, and she has successfully managed a number of funded research projects in these areas. It was for this work that she was awarded the Sigma Theta Tau Honor Society distinguished nurse researcher award (2000) and a Fellowship of the Royal College of Nursing (2002). She is widely published in her field, with her books being translated into other languages. She sits on a number of editorial boards and committees including the International Association for Human Caring and the Florence Nightingale Foundation.

Kathleen Galvin PhD BSc (Hons) RGN

Kathleen is Head of Research and Professor of Health Research at the Institute of Health and Community Studies, Bournemouth University where she has a lead role in developing and supporting the school's research strategy and its development. Her research interests include user perspectives of health and social care; the development of nursing roles; the use and development of methodologies to explore and advance practice; and the use of qualitative, multimethod and action research in evaluating health and social care services. Kathleen has led a range of research projects including an exploration of home-based therapy for children with brain injury; a follow-up study of drug-using offenders who accessed treatment via an arrest referral scheme; an evaluation of citizens advice in general practice; and an action research investigation of facilitating change in a primary care nursing team.

Brendan McCormack DPhil BSc (Hons) PGCEA RNT RMN RGN MILT

Brendan is Director of Nursing Research, Practice Development & Clinical Education, Royal Group of Hospitals, Belfast and University of Ulster at Jordanstown. He began his nursing career as a psychiatric nurse in the Republic of Ireland where he developed particular interests in older people with mental health needs. He then trained as a general nurse in Reading, Berkshire, England and soon after completed a Postgraduate Certificate in the Education of Adults. Having worked as a job-share charge nurse in general surgery Brendan was appointed as the Clothworkers Foundation Clinical Lecturer. He completed a Doctorate in Philosophy at the University of Oxford's Department of Educational Studies, focusing on the autonomy of older people in hospitals, and became head of Practice Development in Oxfordshire Community Health NHS Trust. In his current post, Brendan is Director of Research, Practice Development and Clinical Education in the Royal Hospitals, Belfast. He has recently been elected Chair of the UK Practice Development Forum (a UK-wide network of practice developers) and has written extensively on gerontological nursing and practice development, serving on a number of editorial boards, policy committees and development groups in these areas.

Hugh McKenna PhD BSc (Hons) RMN RGN FFN RCSI

Hugh is Head of School of Nursing, University of Ulster, Northern Ireland Ulster. Hugh has over sixteen years' experience in general and psychiatric nursing. He has over one hundred publications, many of which relate to the development of and testing of knowledge in nursing. He is the Northern Ireland Editor of the *All Ireland Journal of Nursing and Midwifery* and Associate Editor of *Quality and Safety in Health Care* and the *International Journal of Nursing Studies*. He is also an editorial board member of four other international journals. He sits on several regional, national and international committees. He is treasurer of the US-based International Nurse Doctorate Education Network, Vice

Chair of the Northern Ireland Health and Social Care Research Forum and Chair of the Northern Ireland Department of Health and Social Services Nursing R&D Committee. He is a member of a number of scientific committees, the Higher Education Funding Council's Research Assessment Exercise Panel and steering group member of the UK Mental Health Nursing Research Network (Oxford). He has a number of honours, including a Fellowship from the Royal College of Surgeons in Ireland. He is currently involved in post-doctoral research into skill mix, the health promotion needs of young people and an international collaborative study entitled Perceptions of Unit Quality. He is married with two children and lives in Jordanstown, Northern Ireland.

Ann McMahon MSc RN

Ann has held the post of RCN Research and Development Adviser since 1995. Through a stakeholder consultation exercise she developed the RCN's R&D strategy and established the RCN R&D Co-ordinating Centre at the University of Manchester. From here she directs a programme of work which influences research commissioning agendas, develops and makes accessible to nurses support for R&D activity and disseminates knowledge and information to nurses to inform policy and practice decision making. She supports the work of the RCN's Research Society and is a member of the Scientific Committee of the RCN's annual international nursing research conference where she endeavours continually to improve the quality of the conference and increase the transparency of the scientific process. She has an extensive portfolio of publications in professional journals and presentations at local, regional, national and international levels. She is currently registered for a PhD in the Management School at Lancaster University where she is examining innovations in health service delivery from a critical perspective.

Rob Newell PhD BSc RGN RMN RNT

Professor of Nursing Research, School of Health Studies, University of Bradford, Rob is a nurse behaviour therapist by speciality and has been active in this field for twenty years, principally in behavioural medicine. He has been Professor of Nursing Research at the University of Bradford since January 2001. Before taking up this post, he led the Research Support Team for Nurses, Midwives and Health Visitors for Northern and Yorkshire Region, a research capacity building team. His chief area of research interest is in the area of disfigurement, about which he has researched and published widely, but he is also active in collaborative research and development with clinical practitioners, principally in the area of evaluation of nursing practice. Rob has an interest in evidence-based practice and clinical effectiveness and is the editor of the journal *Clinical Effectiveness in Nursing*, the aim of which is once again to examine the effectiveness or otherwise of nursing interventions with patients.

Carol Picard PhD RN CS

Carol is Professor, University of Massachusetts, Massachusetts. Her programme of research examines health as expanding consciousness and the importance of embodied meaning and its expression using creative movement. She has also examined the use of storytelling and sharing of accounts among family members as a way of healing grief and the experience of cancer survivorship for nurses. Carol is Vice-President of Sigma Theta Tau International and President of the International Association for Human Caring. As a result of this work she has vast experience and expertise in developing international networks. She is widely published and is an international member of the editorial board of NT *Research*.

Anne Marie Rafferty DPhil BSc RN FRCN

Director, Centre for Policy in Nursing Research, London School of Hygiene & Tropical Medicine, Anne Marie Rafferty graduated BSc (Soc Sci) in Nursing Studies from Edinburgh University before working as a staff nurse at the Royal Infirmary of Edinburgh. She then moved to the University of Nottingham to the Nursing Studies Unit as a staff nurse and studied part time for an MPhil (Surgery). Switching fields she graduated with a DPhil in Modern History from the University of Oxford before returning to Nottingham University where she was appointed as a lecturer in Nursing Studies. Anne-Marie then spent a year in the US at the University of Pennsylvania as a Harkness Fellow before being appointed Director in 1995 of the then newly formed Centre for Policy in Nursing Research at the London School of Hygiene and Tropical Medicine. She is widely published and closely involved, through the Department of Health and other agencies, in promoting and supporting nursing research.

Sabi Redwood MA RGN RSCN

Sabi is Senior Lecturer in Research, Institute of Health and Community Studies, Bournemouth University. In her current post she has been appointed to lead, support and teach research curricula across a range of undergraduate and post-graduate programmes in health and social care education. Her Doctorate in Education at the University of East Anglia is in progress. Her interests in learning and teaching include open, flexible learning and the role of culture in learning relationships. She also provides leadership and supervision for a range of educational projects exploring alternative models of student practice placements, support and supervision, educational roles in practice and the introduction of cultural competence into the curriculum. She is currently working on an evaluation of the roles of nurse consultant, lecturer practitioner and practice educator.

Michael Traynor PhD MA HV RN

Senior Lecturer, Centre for Policy in Nursing Research London School of Hygiene & Tropical Medicine. Michael read English Literature at Cambridge, then completed general nursing and health visiting training. After working as a health visitor in London he moved to Australia where he was a researcher for the South Australian Health Commission. In 1991 he started work in the Daphne Heald Research Unit at the Royal College of Nursing in London and undertook a three-year examination of nursing morale and values in the wake of the 1991 NHS reforms. Drawing on his background in literature, his PhD examined the language and rhetoric employed by nurses and their managers. He presently works as lecturer at the Centre for Policy in Nursing Research at the London School of Hygiene & Tropical Medicine. His interests include applying discourse analysis and poststructuralist approaches to nursing policy and health care issues.

Part I

Policy and Professional Considerations

1 The context of clinical research: Policy and professionalism

Veronica Bishop and Dawn Freshwater

A service with ambitions is one that invests in the future NHS through research and development, and which ensures that the most effective practice is used throughout the NHS (DoH 1996)

The aim of this chapter is to provide a brief critique of the modern health service in the UK and to highlight the need for nursing to develop a genuine culture of research that can enable the profession to deliver research-oriented practice. It is argued that this will not only raise the standard of care but will also develop the level of professional knowledge, credibility and accountability of practitioners. Links between research and clinical governance and evidence-based practice are made; moreover this chapter also seeks to outline the development of research within nursing and the wider implications for the position of nursing within the academy, within health care and in society.

Introduction

The creation of the National Health Service (NHS) in 1948 was a remarkable achievement, offering its services free at the point of delivery and financed from general taxation. The dominant biomedical model of health care, which underpinned the introduction of the NHS, has predominated for most of the twentieth century, with minor tweaking or organisational experimentation. The major resource implications concomitant with the provision of free care have made the NHS into something of a political football. While the last two governments have both sought to create changes which reflect their ideology, Wilmot (2003:42) notes that neither government has noticeably achieved significant change in the wider society, and in that respect Bevan retains the prize!

Nursing in the NHS

Despite nursing constituting the largest professional group involved in health care the prestige and influence that such predominance might assume is not there. The reasons for this, such as medical dominance and power systems, gender and class issues are well documented throughout the range of nursing literature. Indeed it is the narrative that nursing has been brought up with. However, a combination of many factors, including increased diversity of health care options, increased emphasis on health education and promotion, the more open introduction and promotion of complementary therapies and a more aware, educated and indeed litigious population which demands greater diversity and self-involvement, is effecting more change that any single government. These changes offer major opportunities for nurses. Such changes can be met with a great deal of optimism by the nursing and midwifery professions. Influenced by its less traditionally hidebound colleagues in the United States and Australia, nursing has developed a more autonomous role since the early 1970s. Salvage (1992) attributes much of this changed perception of nursing to the strengthening of the women's movement and to the challenge to the assumption that nursing is subordinate to medicine, set against improved standards of education. While the contribution of male nurses to the gender debate is barely noted by authors beyond the fact that the largest percentage of top jobs in nursing have traditionally been held by men, certainly the move of nursing and midwifery education into institutions of higher education has had a major impact on students' perceptions of their future roles and contribution. Qualified nurses and midwives are now far more assertive in their clinical areas, and many seek to be involved at high-level management. While it would be far too optimistic to say that the 'glass ceiling' is broken, there is much evidence (female nurses at board level, female ministers and chief executives in business and health care) to suggest that it is within touching distance. There are, none the less, challenges associated with the move of education of all the health care professions into higher education. Changes in patterns of health care delivery, the increased autonomy of individual health care professionals and the need to utilise limited resources in an ever-demanding system, have led to greater multidisciplinary working and to the growth of schools of health rather than schools of nursing and midwifery. Political correctness almost demands that we embrace this with enthusiasm. Indeed many colleagues truly enjoy the breadth of expertise that such arrangements can offer. However, if nursing, along with many other professions, struggles with a theory–practice gap, as Wilmot (2003) and many others contend (see, for example, Freshwater and Rolfe, 2001; Rolfe, Freshwater and Jasper, 2001) then it is crucial that professional knowledge and the development of the academy of nursing have a strong focus. Wilmot goes on to suggest that while nursing necessarily seeks to accommodate a wide range of knowledge and expertise, it renders itself open to criticism of being over-inclusive and possibly incoherent. Despite this observation Wilmot (2003:101) argues that 'if the health and social care professions are propelled toward convergence in the coming years ... in the case of nursing it is particularly important that its open and flexible approach to health care is not lost in the process of homogenisation'. It is our view that if professional nursing is not to fall into a generic health care worker abyss, taking up all tasks dropped by other team members who are more clear as to their unique contribution to health care services, it must clarify its role and have evidence to support its value. This is not an easy task – if it was it would have been accomplished decades ago, modified to match progress.

The importance of research and development in the NHS presents a major challenge to nurses. Without research-based evidence to support nursing practice and to underpin standards there are no criteria for care provision and few substantive arguments for qualified staff. Bishop and Scott (2001) contend that the infrastructure to support either well-constructed or well-conducted research in nursing is not, as yet, sufficient. They go on to say that while it is not necessarily the role of all qualified nurses to undertake research it is essential for all practitioners to be able to access and understand research findings for the purpose of monitoring, evaluating and improving practice (Bishop and Scott, 2001). It is crucial, as Rafferty et al. point out in Chapter 2, to build the capacity and capability of nurses to seek out and achieve ownership of research findings in order to ensure that nursing practice is substantiated by the best available evidence. What constitutes 'best evidence' will not be debated in this chapter but is considered in detail by Freshwater in Chapter 4. It is nearly three decades since Chater (1975) argued that patient care should be founded on defensible, research-based findings, that is, underpinned by scientific principles. Additionally it has been stated that not to base nursing practice on research is unethical (Styles, 1982). However, it has also been contested that one of the biggest challenges facing nursing is the development of the profession through application of research findings (Freshwater and Broughton, 2001; Tierney, 1998; Le May, Mulhall and Alexander, 1998).

Nursing and research

Since Briggs (1972) stated that nursing should be a research-based profession, career opportunities have gradually developed for nurses, sometimes outside the nursing professions and more recently from within. Major policy initiatives such as the publication of *Making a Difference* (DoH, 1999), which espouses the implementation of joint appointments in order to bridge the theory–practice and research gap and the introduction of nurse consultant posts, have placed research career pathways firmly on the map of professional development. However, this was not always the case.

In 1988 the House of Lords Select Committee on Science and Technology reported on *Priorities in Medical Research*. This committee was formed in part as a result of the apparent decline in international standing of UK science and technology. The committee reported that morale was low and funding inadequate within the medical research community and that the NHS was run with little awareness of the needs of research or what it had to offer. As a result of these findings a director of research and development was appointed at the Department of Health who was to announce a new research and development strategy, *Research for Health* (DoH, 1991). This strategy was designed to strengthen the commitment to systematic enquiry, evaluation and knowledge-based practice throughout the NHS. The formal response to this from nursing was published in 1992 (DoH, 1992) and included 37 recommendations. All of them were highly relevant, but the authors of the document could be considered somewhat naïve in presenting such a large number of issues to be addressed; indeed it could be argued that the report achieved very little and that any subsequent progress was barely attributable to its content. Much of this lack of progress may be laid at the door of the overall research and development policy, which rigidly prescribed areas suitable for research funding, all of which were appropriate for qualitative lines of enquiry.

Lorentzon expressed well the difficulties of obtaining funding for nursing research when funding was heavily dependent on particular types of proposals, saying that 'the diffuse nature of most nurse–patient interactions makes it difficult to measure the effect of interventions in a systematic manner. Quantitative aspects of nursing care are not easily evaluated except in terms of general patient satisfaction' (p. 825). Policy initiatives leading to and following the Task Force Report are described by Rafferty et al. in Chapter 2, but despite significant progress in medical research and development strategies it is argued that nursing research and development strategies throughout the UK remain poorly structured to date, with just a few pockets of excellence. However, as Rafferty et al. highlight, there are several initiatives currently being developed which should present a much healthier picture in the near future and which certainly offer much to build on. None the less it is noted in the recent publication on Scottish nursing and midwifery strategic research that 'moving forward presents many challenges and some tough choices as nurses and midwives explore how best to maximise opportunities within the current environment' (Scottish Executive, 2002:41).

The term 'clinical research' is common terminology in medical practice but has not yet been accepted as normal within nursing parlance. Nursing research is often perceived as investigation into nurses rather than into the care they provide. In fact nursing research may reach into any sphere pertaining to patient care and nursing interactions, professional roles and workforce issues and, just as importantly, the development of nursing knowledge. The dramatic changes in nursing care resulting from high patient turnover, new demands in the community, altered arrangements in service provision and, not least, major developments in technology and pharmacology, have changed what is expected of qualified practitioners, and areas to be researched must reflect these changes. It is the provision of professional, knowledgeable care that must identify the nursing profession (Bishop, 2001). McKenna and Mason (1998) maintain that the goal of nursing research should be to carry out rigorous, systematic enquiry designed to make significant contributions to knowledge. They go further to state that such knowledge should impact positively on the physical, mental and social well-being of the population. The argument that nursing has a series of key roles to play in health service research at strategic and operational levels, while retaining the flexibility to focus on issues and phenomena that are predominately the concern of the nursing profession, is well made.

There are obvious difficulties in separating issues which have a direct impact on patients and clients. In the rush to show that as professionals we don't baulk at a challenge, we have striven to mimic or to adapt models of investigation which are well established in the medical disciplines as well as to develop new lines of enquiry. Some of the models of investigation used are less than satisfactory in the search for nursing outcomes but are pursued because funding bodies deem them superior and thus essential. A great deal of debate has developed on the values of qualitative and quantitative paradigms (Blaxter, Hughes and Tight, 2001; Rolfe, et al., 2001; Webb, 1996) and anyone considering a career in research will find themselves at some point enmeshed in these! None the less much good work has been replicated using different approaches but, regrettably, despite the profession seeking to expand its body of knowledge by researching and identifying clinically effective practices, the impact of that knowledge on health care currently founders. Implementation can be best described as patchy and, while the reasons for this have been discussed widely, as yet career opportunities, pressure of time on practitioners, limited resources for practitioners and short-sighted managers have all conspired, in many localities, to keep this as a major issue to be addressed.

Stevens (1997) suggests that, while many clinical practitioners and academics are actively promoting the concept of clinical effectiveness through nursing research and development, and despite the raised awareness from broader educational programmes, we have failed as a profession to make clinical effectiveness a part of everyday business. She goes on to suggest that a national strategic framework is needed to help nursing respond to the opportunities presented by evidence-based practice, which at some level appears to conflict with what other authors term practitioner-based approaches to research, but may be necessary for the debate to be taken seriously (Freshwater and Rolfe, 2001; Jarvis, 2000). Keighley (2003) suggests that 'a major concern has been the development of specialist nurse education in the European Union ... which has led to a series of reviews being conducted into how specialist nursing is developing'. Stevens sees specialisation as a potential divisor and considers that serious deficits exist which militate against nurses' ability to influence change. The challenge to which Stevens refers is, perhaps, the ability of the profession to maintain a united front in the political arena while struggling for recognition in specific clinical or academic spheres. She states that the art is to recognise the need for specialisation while not allowing it to lead to segregation or professional insularity.

There is no doubting the truth of the saying 'divide and rule', and nursing as a whole has not shown itself as a force to be reckoned with in the way that medical colleagues have, despite the disparity in numbers between the two professions. The need for 'political nous' is the clarion call of Salvage (1998) who wonders if, in the rush to embrace nursing research and evidence-based practice, we are losing the plot. She points out that, as with most policy developments, the research and development initiatives mix altruism with pragmatism. Nursing, in her view, needs to be fully alert in its attempts to influence the research and development agenda and to 'avoid selling out' in our attempts to 'buy in'. This is a view she shares with Maggs (1997) who highlights the fact that experimental research, which is predominately reductionist, ignores the philosophical basis of nursing and of caring.

The lack of a cohesive strategy in nursing research, despite the great optimism for change with a new government in 1997, is well documented in the professional journals, and cogent arguments were made for the reversal of this state of affairs (Rafferty, Bond and Traynor, 2000; *NT* Research Symposium 1998; Kitson et al., 1997; DoH, 1992). In September 2001 a meeting was held in York between the Director of Research and Development at the Department of Health and some key players in the field of nursing research and the NHS. It was agreed that, despite considerable progress in nursing research in recent years, current arrangements failed to maximise the nursing contribution to research and development. Also, while some of the constraints reflected lack of professional confidence and co-ordination, significant institutional barriers have constrained development of both capacity and capability. The recommendations of this report are discussed in the appropriate chapters of this book, and ways in which the professional can both use and contribute to the developing strategy for good nursing and therapeutic research are clearly signposted.

Having sketched out the overall context of nursing research in policy terms it is essential to ensure the reader is familiar with the terminology or language in current use across all the disciplines, and it is to this that we will now turn our attention.

Clinical effectiveness

Clinical effectiveness can be defined as:

> The extent to which specific clinical interventions, when deployed in the field for a particular patient or population, do what they are intended to do, that is, maintain and improve health and secure the greatest possible health gain from the available resources. (NHS, 1996:3)

This definition is seen by many to be another term for cost-effectiveness and as such many professions are adapting it to sit more comfortably with their own professional philosophies. The Royal College of Nursing (RCN) for example uses the definition 'Applying the best available knowledge for research, clinical expertise and patient preferences to achieve optimum processes and outcomes of care for patients' (RCN, 1998:3). In this definition the Royal College of Nursing draws attention to the variation between standards and levels of care with the purpose of achieving excellence in clinical practice (Freshwater and Broughton, 2001).

We have already mentioned several times the concept of evidence-based practice, a further term that is currently well rehearsed in everyday health care practices. The literature and diversity of opinions around evidence-based practice is almost overwhelming. As Freshwater and Broughton (2001:67) note, 'There are many definitions of evidence based practice, evidence based health care, evidence based nursing and the forerunner of them all – evidence based medicine, some of them more "user friendly" than others'. Many of the definitions are derived from evidence-based medicine. Sackett, Rosenberg, Gray et al. (1996), for example, write of the 'conscientious, explicit and judicious use of current best evidence' (p. 62). This definition is based on the notion of best medical practice, which, as Freshwater and Broughton (2000) point out, has been determined by the use of randomised controlled trials, which are often inappropriate for the investigation of issues into nursing and associated therapies. As Marks-Maran (1999) remarks, nursing is not a linear process and, while nursing may attempt to order its processes, the world of the patient can be chaotic; as a consequence, nursing must develop an evidence base that is in keeping with its own philosophies and practices. Thus, nursing practice and indeed nursing research has to date been defined by the modernist rationalistic model that is the dominant paradigm of the medical model.

The data for evidence-based practice can be sought from a variety of sources including research studies, literature searches and meta-analyses, as well as from regular audit material, expert opinions and of course the users and carers of the services themselves. Critical skills are necessary to assess and evaluate the wealth of available evidence and its relevance to clinical practice. (The development of critical appraisal and other related skills is dealt with in significant detail in Chapter 4, as is the debate surrounding what constitutes evidence.)

The gulf between research and practice, not only in nursing but also in all health-related disciplines in health care, is longstanding. In a move to bridge that gulf in the UK the statement 'A service with ambitions is one that invests in the future NHS through research and development, which ensures that the most effective practice is used throughout the NHS' (DoH, 1996) has heralded a movement claiming to highlight evidence-based practice. The drive for evidence-based practice, while introduced for reasons of economics rather than health, offers the opportunity to redress that imbalance and bridge the gap constructively. There is a downside, in that only outcomes of care are measured and often processes are ignored. A greatly respected worldwide expert in the quality in health care, Donabedian (1988), stressed the equal importance of process with outcome. As much of nursing is process rather than an easily defined intervention, a model of evidence-based practice which ignores, because of the difficulty in measurement, the philosophical basis of nursing disregards the activities of the largest health care workforce. In particular it disregards any notions of therapeutic environments (Freshwater, 2002), a loss in our view to the philosophical underpinnings of research and to those issues which drive research in health care. This is particularly relevant to nursing, which has a basis of knowledgeable caring rather than cut-and-dried interventions. A further criticism of evidence-based practice is that in many studies which lend themselves to experimental or randomised controlled trials, the questions asked are limited to the method, and exclusion and inclusion criteria are necessarily so rigorous that the application of the results is limited to a similar population. None the less the culture created by the introduction of evidence-based practice is to be welcomed as one of raising questions about potential improvement to patient care. Both evidence-based practice and clinical effectiveness are closely embedded in the move towards clinical governance.

Clinical governance

Clinical governance was first discussed in the Department of Health document *A First Class Service – Quality in the New NHS* (DoH, 1998:2) and was also a feature of the NHS Plan (DoH, 2000). It can be defined as 'The process by which each part of the NHS quality assures its clinical decisions. Backed by a new statutory duty of quality it will introduce a system of continuous improvement into the operation of the whole NHS' (DoH 1998:9).

The term governance means the direction and control of the actions, affairs, policies and functions of an organisation (*Collins English Dictionary*, 1982), therefore prefacing the term with 'clinical' we can determine that clinical activity will form the basis of all future actions and developments and will underpin the future of the NHS (Scott, 1999:38). Clinical governance then is primarily concerned with standards and the dissemination of best evidence. This necessitates that nurses, in order to contribute fully to the health care agenda, become more politically aware and astute. Opportunities exist for their involvement in decision making at policy level. The bottom line in clinical governance, and for those involved in its processes, is the need for a real understanding of the research processes, particularly in relation to clinical effectiveness. Forming part of a ten-year programme of work, clinical governance has initiated an innovative approach to ownership of clinical decision making and, since this national initiative was launched, several bodies have been set up to oversee its implementation.

Key national standards organisations are:

- National Institute for Clinical Excellence (NICE)
- Commission for Health Improvement (CHI)
- National Institute for Mental Health Excellence (NIMHE).

These statutory bodies are involved in ensuring the local delivery of high-quality clinical services through such frameworks as the National Service Frameworks (NSF) and local Health Improvement Plans (HImPs).

In March 2001 the Government issued a research governance framework for health and social care. Research governance sets the standards and the mechanisms to deliver and monitor them, thus improving research quality and safeguarding the public. This was largely as a result of high media exposure of unethical practices in medical practice and research but also a reflection of the realisation that greater co-ordination and shared ethics were essential in a massive researchable population to prevent human exploitation, duplication of effort and misuse of limited resources. The framework, which is available on the Department of Health updated website reflects consultation between the NHS, the Department of Health and key players in the health care and social care sectors. It defines the broad principles of good research governance and is seen as key to ensuring that health and social care research is conducted to high scientific and ethical standards.

Any organisation participating in research must now have a system in place to ensure that all ongoing research is logged as having senior approval and ethics committee approval. This does not just apply to research undertaken with patients and clients but embraces research across the spectrum of the NHS. This includes projects by students, staff questionnaires and other smaller studies that previously had sometimes been allowed to progress 'on the nod' and were never formally presented to research ethics committees. The reasoning behind this move to formalise all studies is sound – not only will it prevent over-taxing specific populations (an example of this occurred in the 1980s when HIV/Aids patients were inundated with requests for information in the drive to tailor services to their needs) but also it should ensure that data derived from small studies are where possible aggregated, thus adding to the overall development of a knowledge base.

What should be implicit in any framework to support high-quality research, and should ideally be made explicit, is the link between the researcher and his or her supervisor and/or peer review body. Many researchers, of all disciplines, while academically qualified, are expected to work without supervision or external academic advice and this is not conducive to well-critiqued work. For example, the current focus on primary care research will need to address this in order to prevent research questions, and findings, being developed in isolation from other services and disciplines. An example of a recent community-based project that aimed to develop its services in collaboration with secondary and tertiary care is the implementation of the Diana Children's Community Nursing Team funded by the Department of Health (Danvers et al., 2002), which sought to implement a new service for children with life limiting illness.

As part of the service implementation an evaluation study was conducted in order to highlight the added value of the new service for the children, their families, the Diana nurses themselves and, as importantly, the other services which are closely linked to the care of such children. An external team was commissioned to undertake the evaluation, which included members of the Diana Children's Community Team and external evaluators in the shape of experienced researchers, academic advisors, expert consultants across a variety of services that is, paediatrician, paediatric social worker, a general practitioner and a user of the service. The practitioner/researcher leading the evaluation team was an experienced sick children's nurse working within secondary care and she continued to manage a caseload throughout the two-year duration of the study. External supervision was provided by a researcher/practitioner, that is, someone with expertise in managing and completing complex evaluation projects but who also maintained a clinical practice, although not in the specialist field of children's nursing. Importantly, someone working across primary and secondary care carried out the evaluation itself and, in addition, staff across primary, secondary and tertiary care contributed to the analysis and evaluation of the project.

What does all this mean for research in contemporary nursing?

Research in any health discipline is about supporting excellence in care. Excellence is generally hard won, particularly in health care with so many conflicting issues, but always within reach if the thinking is clear and the carer committed. Asked recently what she considered essential to be an excellent researcher, one author responded 'enthusiasm and discipline'. One without the other could be disastrous. Despite the less than rosy historical policy picture presented above, the reader has the option participating in an exciting challenge rather than a course to be avoided. Nursing is a relatively new profession, and should be heartened by what has been achieved to date. But it is not a time to stand still, nor can it ever be in health care. There are wonderful opportunities to really push the boundaries of nursing and to achieve at a personal level what might have been thought of as impossible – examples of this are cited in Chapter 7 which looks at some individual careers in research.

In summary, then, there are three ways to consider involvement in research in contemporary nursing, which are outlined below. However, it is important to note here that we also believe that research is a part of every practitioner's role and if using a practitioner/researcher model then each practitioner is engaging in all three of these levels simultaneously, with one perhaps being more foreground at any one time.

Levels of research involvement

1. At a general level, ensure that your practice is evidence based, where good evidence exists; to be able to differentiate between good research and the not so good.

2. At a facilitate level, ensure that those who have an aptitude for research are supported and encouraged; feed their work into the overall organisation.
3. At a personal/professional development level, where research is undertaken.

First level: General practice

If health care that is relevant and appropriate is to be given to service users, the practitioners providing that service must be knowledgeable and up to date. Health care is dynamic, always changing in the light of new evidence, new diagnoses and new treatments. In nursing there is, as stated earlier, a statutory requirement for the practitioner to be well versed in their area of care, and this is certainly part and parcel of the ethos of nursing. However, strategies for developing clinical practice must not be advanced in a vacuum; in other words, policy must be informed by practice and, just as importantly, practitioners must take the time to stand back and reflect on their approaches. Different trusts offer varying opportunities for research-minded staff. Library facilities, online access and research facilitators are unfortunately not yet in place across all of the UK, and it must be admitted that sometimes lip-service alone serves the eager would-be investigator. Be aware of the variations when applying for a post, consider important factors such as basic online library access and if it is unavailable then you may need to look elsewhere. That said, there are many organisations that have good infrastructures set up to support the development of research, but the practitioners do not make the time to utilise them.

Research mindedness and evidence-based care have to be worked at, and time has to be woven into the timetable for any degree of success. One of the most helpful and legitimate methods of taking time for yourself is through clinical supervision and critical reflection (Rolfe et al., 2001; Bishop, 1998; Binnie and Titchen, 1995) and of course by reading professional journals and attending conferences, workshops and other forms of continuing professional development.

Research mindedness is a matter of taking a questioning approach to your work and to the work of others. This does not mean criticism, but rather a reflective stroll around the issue being discussed, looking at it from a different perspective, particularly from the patient's view, and re-evaluating the outcome to date; a mental camera, if you like, that takes snaps from many angles. A good example of the need to have done this is described by McMahon (2002) who describes the difficulty a friend had in persuading nurses to review their treatment of an elderly lady with continence difficulties and venous leg ulcers. Determined to use the well-evidenced three-layer pressure bandage they omitted to take on board the fact that the lady was immobilised by the bandages and as a consequence was unable to appease her bladder. Soaked bandages are not indicative of holistic thinking and a questioning approach.

Second level: Facilitation

Clinical nurses need access to research-based information and, most importantly, access to knowledgeable staff to support them in their enquiries. Staff who have a research facilitation role need to be sensitive to the degree of expertise of the practitioner and how to strengthen this. Developing a research culture is central to successful implementation of research finding, to questioning practices and to improving health care services. Collaboration with accessible academic institutions should be made, focusing on pertinent clinical issues and harnessing both clinical and academic expertise. A research facilitator should know no barriers and seek novices, experts, information and support from any and every crevice. It is not a post for anyone less than totally committed, but one with wonderful opportunities.

Third level: Dedicated researcher

Education of any kind offers choices which were possibly hitherto unlikely, and extending formal education to undertaking a research degree can only increase the student's view of his or her world and the choices within it. As this publication goes to print there are national and local strategies being developed which will ensure that nurse research and nurse researchers become a part of the wide health care agenda. The political will is bending to the ear of our increasing knowledge and expertise, with career paths in nursing research beginning to reflect this more widely. More importantly there is now a move from fixed focus on education and organisational research subjects to recognition that nursing research must also address clinical issues – a real challenge in terms of what methods of investigation to use. Given the small amount of evidence we have in nursing compared to the vast amount of care that we provide the research agenda for our profession is enormous.

Conclusion

At every level there is an opportunity to make a change for the better, to achieve satisfaction in work and to contribute to one of the most important agendas for the universe – quality health care. The following chapters offer insights into how the individual practitioner may approach these challenges with knowledge, confidence and optimism.

Key points

- The main focus of nursing research is to underpin and support the nursing profession in its drive to develop highly knowledgeable staff to provide appropriate care.
- Research is part of every practitioner's role.
- The process of nursing is as valid as its outcome.
- Clinical effectiveness must be part of everyday business.

References

Binnie, A. and Titchen, A. (1995) The art of clinical supervision. *British Journal of Nursing*, **4**: 327–34.

Bishop, V. and Scott, I. (eds) (2001) *Challenges in Clinical Practice. Professional developments in nursing.* Basingstoke: Palgrave – now Palgrave Macmillan.

Bishop, V. (ed.) (1998) *Clinical Supervision in Practice*. London: Macmillan – now Palgrave Macmillan.

Bishop, V. (2001) Professional development and clinical supervision. In *Challenges in Clinical Practice. Professional developments in nursing*. Basingstoke: Palgrave – now Palgrave Macmillan.

Bishop, V. and Scott, I. (2001) Introduction. In Bishop, V. and Scott, I. (eds) *Challenges in Clinical Practice. Professional developments in nursing*. Basingstoke: Palgrave – now Palgrave Macmillan.

Blaxter, L., Hughes, C. and Tight, C. (2001) *How to research*, 2nd edn, Buckinghamshire: Open University Press.

Briggs, A. (1972) *Committee on Nursing*. Cmnd. 5115, London: HMSO.

Chater, S. (1975) *Understanding research in nursing*. Geneva: WHO.

Collins English Dictionary (1982) Collins: London.

Danvers, L., Freshwater, D., Cheater, F. and Wilson, A. (2002) An Evaluation of the Diana Children's Community Nursing Service for Children with Life Limiting Illness. *NTResearch*. 7(3): 187–98.

DoH (Department of Health) (1991) *Research for Health: A research and development strategy for the NHS*. London: HMSO.

DoH (Department of Health) (1992) R*eport of the task force on the strategy for research in nursing, midwifery and health visiting*. London: HMSO.

DoH (Department of Health) (1996) *The National Health Service – Service with Ambitions*. White Paper, Nov Cmnd 3425. London: The Stationary Office.

DoH (Department of Health) (1998) *A First Class Service: Quality in the New NHS*. Wetherby: DoH. www.doh.gov.uk/newnhs/qualsum.htm

DoH (Department of Health) (1999) *Making a difference. Strengthening the Nursing, Midwifery and Health Visiting Contribution to Health and Healthcare*. London: DoH.

DoH (Department of Health) (2000) *The NHS Plan*. London: DoH.

DoH (Department of Health) (2001) *Towards a Strategy for Nursing Research and Development. Proposals for Action*. London: DoH.

Donebedian, A. (1988) Inquiry 25 173.

Freshwater, D. (ed.) (2002) *Therapeutic Nursing*. London: Sage.

Freshwater, D. and Broughton, R. (2001) Research and Evidence Based Practice. In Bishop, V. and Scott, I. (eds) (2001) *Challenges in Clinical Practice. Professional developments in nursing*. Basingstoke: Palgrave – now Palgrave Macmillan.

Freshwater, D. and Rolfe, G. (2001) Critical Reflexivity: A politically and ethically engaged research method for nursing. *NTResearch*, 6(1): 526–37.

House of Lords Select Committee on Science and Technology (1988) *Priorities in Medical Research*. 1st Report. London: HMSO.

Jarvis, A. (2000) The practitioner-researcher in nursing. *Nurse Education Today*, **20**: 30–5.

Keighley, T. (2003) Nursings Role in Shaping European Health Policy. In Tadd, W. (ed.) *Professional Issues in Nursing: Perspectives from Europe*. Basingstoke: Palgrave Macmillan.

Kitson, A., McMahon, A., Rafferty, A. and Scott, L. (1997) On developing an agenda to influence policy in health care research for effective nursing: A description of a national R&D Priority Setting Exercise. *Nursing Times Research*, 2(5): 323–34.

Le May, A., Mulhall, A. and Alexander, C. (1998) Bridging the research–practice gap: exploring the research cultures of practitioners and managers. *Journal of Advanced Nursing*, 28(2): 428–37.

Lorentzon, M. (1995) Multidisciplinary collaboration: lifeline or drowning pool for nurse researchers. *Journal of Advanced Nursing*, 22(5): 825.

McKenna, H. and Mason, C. (1998) Nursing and the wider R&D agenda: Influence and contribution. *NTResearch*, 3(2): 108–15.

McMahon, A. (2002) Let's get critical. Guest editorial. *Nursing Times Research*, 7(5): 322–3.

Maggs, C. (1997) Research and the nursing agenda. Confronting what we believe nursing to be. *NTResearch*, 2(5): 321–2.

Marks-Maran, D. (1999) Reconstructing nursing: evidence, artistry and the curriculum. *Nurse Education Today*, 3–11.

NHS (National Health Service Executive) (1996) *Promoting Clinical Effectiveness: A framework for action in and through the NHS*. Leeds: NHSE.

NT Research Symposium (1998) Proceedings. *Nursing Times Research*, 3(1): 8–28.

Payne, J.P. (1999) Supervisors' comments. In Bishop, V. (ed.) *Working towards a research degree*. Emap Publications: London.

Rafferty, A.M., Bond, S. and Traynor, M. (2000) Does Nursing, Midwifery and Health Visiting need a research council? *NTResearch*, 5: 325–35.

RCN (Royal College of Nursing) (1998) *Edlines*. London: RCN.

Rolfe, G., Freshwater, D. and Jasper, M. (2001) *Critical reflection for nursing and the helping professions: A users guide*. Basingstoke: Palgrave – now Palgrave Macmillan.

Sackett, D.L., Rosenberg, W., Gray, J.A.M., Haynes, R.B. and Richardson, W.S. (1996) Evidence based medicine: what it is and what it isn't. *British Medical Journal*, 312: 71–2.

Salvage, J. (1992) The New Nursing: Empowering patients or empowering nurses? In Robinson, J., Gray, A. and Elkan, R. (eds). *Policy Issues in Nursing*. Buckingham: Open University Press.

Salvage, J. (1998) Evidence based practice: a mixture of motives? *NTResearch*, 3(6): 406–18.

Scott, I. (1999) Clinical Governance, a framework for practice. In Bishop, V. and Scott, I. (eds.). *Challenges in Clinical Practice*. Palgrave – now Palgrave Macmillan: Basingstoke.

Stevens, J. (1997) Improving integration between research and practice as a means of developing evidence based health care. *NTResearch*, 2(1): 7–15.

Styles, M.M. (1982) *On nursing toward a new endowment*. St. Louis: C.V. Mosby.

Tierney, A. (1998) The politics of the NHS R&D agenda. *NT Research*, **3**(6): 419–20.
Webb, C. (1996) Action Research. In Cormack, D.F.S. (ed.) *The research process in nursing*, Ch 18. Oxford: Blackwell Scientific.
Wilmot, S. (2003) *Ethics, Power and Policy. The future of nursing in the NHS*. Basingstoke: Palgrave Macmillan.

2 Research and development: Policy and capacity building

Anne Marie Rafferty, Rob Newell and Michael Traynor

This chapter considers the supply and demand factors which drive the case to build capacity in research in nursing, midwifery and health visiting. It reviews the key policy documents and processes and argues that it was not just professional push but also policy pull factors which provided the key catalysts for change. Nursing, midwifery and health visiting roles and responsibilities are increasing in the light of government policies and professional aspirations.

Introduction

An appropriate evidence base is essential for the ability to understand, undertake, commission and implement research and to drive up quality. Research capacity building needs to be integrated into wider strategic plans for the profession as well as Research and Development (R&D) policy *per se*. Establishing a fund to develop high-calibre research is only the beginning of a much longer process of enhancing the analytic power for nursing. Researchers, educators, managers and clinicians need to join forces to build strong communities and strengthen their links with patient and user groups. The investment in nursing and midwifery R&D will have failed if it only ever benefits the professional community. Patient care needs to be part of the 'payback' for investment and an evaluation strategy needs to be evolved which is capable of measuring a range of impacts from the start.

The first cohort of research development awards has recently been announced by the Department of Health and Higher Education Funding Council for England (HEFCE). Both parties agreed to establish a fund to increase the amount of high-quality research related to nursing and allied health professions. Two new award schemes at doctoral and post-doctoral levels for future research leaders have been instituted. The announcements were based on the recommendations of a task group, chaired by Professor Janet Finch, vice-chancellor of Keele University, which looked at how high-quality research relevant to nurses and allied health professions could be better supported. The report found that research in this area was significantly under-funded in comparison with other comparable professions such as teaching, and that the available funding was skewed towards short-term projects. The task group's report presented a clear case for nursing research and a plan for investment to realise its potential (HEFCE, 2001).

While there are reasons to be cheerful about the future of research in nursing and midwifery, and something to celebrate, there is still some way to go to remedy the R&D deficit within the profession. Government reports have consistently noted both the need for greater emphasis on research and development within the National Health Service (NHS), and the need for this research itself to be multidisciplinary has been widely acknowl-edged (DoH, 1994a, 1997a, 1998a). Yet the policy goals, however well intentioned, have rarely translated into action. It must be noted that the largest professions within health care (nursing, midwifery and health visiting), while providing the bulk of health care, experience considerable challenges in their ability to under-stand, undertake, implement and commission research. Nurs-ing, midwifery and health visiting represent the largest single cost item within the largest component of NHS expenditure. It is estimated that three pence in every pound is spent on nursing and yet so little is known about the activities and impact of the largest workforce within the NHS. At one level this could be seen as an irresponsible use of public money. At another it can be viewed as a paradox of policy that in an era obsessed with accountability and the culture of audit such a large part of public expenditure has gone unscrutinised for so long. Much of the push for policy change has come from the professions themselves and has been seen from the outside as being largely self-serving. Arguments for investment have tended to focus on the supply-side of the equation; specifically the scarcity of researchers and the paucity of research. In addition, the notable lack of any uni-fying strategy within government to address the research capacity and evidence-deficit within the NHS and higher education (HE) until recently has meant the issue has occupied a low position on the policy totem pole.

But the mood has changed within government and this is reflected in the strategic alliance between HEFCE and the English Department of Health (DoH) with a pledge towards partnership working to strengthen areas of known weakness. In this sense nursing and midwifery have been helped by an inclusive policy approach designed to embrace allied health professions within its remit. Such a move made it attractive to policy makers since it enables several issues to be tackled with a single solution. In administrative terms it is appealing since it combines utility with economy of effort. Much of the ground-work for the nursing and midwifery action plan was laid at a workshop in York which produced a ground-breaking docu-ment outlining the possible direction a coherent research career structure and strategy might take (DoH, 2000b). This chapter argues that while professional push may be necessary to bring about policy change, policy pull is necessary to secure success. Even after assent has been achieved, further lobbying may be required to ensure the next phase of implementation is secured. But investment carries with it certain responsibilities, and it is important that payback for patients features as a clear focus for evaluation of the programme. In this regard links with patient and user groups could be stronger. There is a great opportunity to develop new methods of commissioning and to evaluate the impact of research, and by doing so to position nursing, mid-wifery and allied health professions in the vanguard of the capacity building field.

The need for access to a sustainable stream of funding for research in nursing, midwifery and health visiting has been recognised for some time (Rafferty, Bond and Traynor, 2000). The argument for the case has been gathering momentum slowly, though thwarted until recently by the preference for multi-disciplinary mainstreaming within R&D policy itself. Now, with capacity building firmly on the agenda for the NHS and HE, the high political profile of the NHS and an array of service and policy initiatives focusing on delivery, the tail-winds of impact seemed to be blowing strongly in nursing's favour. The reasons behind the apparent catalytic convergence between professional and policy agendas have been enumerated by Rafferty, Bond and Traynor (2000). Our aim in this chapter is to:

- map out the main policy drivers for nursing R&D
- consider the implications for capacity building
- comment on what more needs to be done.

Contextualising the case

Two papers stand out as landmarks in recent research policy (DoH, 1993, 2000a) which set out an appropriate direction for the development of research capacity. The first report of the taskforce (DoH, 1993) and the predecessor to the current task group report to the Department of Health (HEFCE, 2001) identified the need for a strategy to secure research activity and, by extension, the evidence base for nursing, midwifery and health visiting. Much of this document was concerned with how capacity for R&D might be built within the professions. Whilst weighing the competing demands for nursing, midwifery and health visiting to become a special case within health service research with its own funding council, or to be integrated and strengthened within the existing research support arrangements, the key notions which emerged from the report were the understanding that nursing, midwifery and health visiting had been disadvantaged in research terms and that this disadvantage should be addressed. The report's recommendations were designed to overcome barriers to the undertaking of research within the professions and to enhance their research performance. Key among its recommendations was a section devoted to research education and training, a central matter for capacity development. These recommendations included:

- addressing lack of research literacy
- additional funding for research training
- research training fellowships and posts in higher education

- research training for clinical staff
- post doctoral fellowships.

More broadly, the report suggested mechanisms whereby the contribution of nursing, midwifery and health visiting to NHS R&D could be broadened and strengthened, for example through recognition of this contribution within the various R&D funding streams and through the location of R&D training within centres of high-quality research supervision.

The second report, *Towards a Strategy for Nursing Research and Development: proposals for Action* (DoH, 2000b) arose from a workshop attended by nursing research leaders in York, UK to explore how a commitment made in *Making a Difference* (DoH, 1999a) might be operationalised. The publication sets out important and familiar barriers to the effectiveness of nursing, midwifery and health visiting as a force in NHS research and also, importantly, notes the findings of a nursing research mapping exercise (Thompson, 2000) and the finding within this of particular pockets of need (for example, concerning research in the areas of elderly care, rehabilitation and primary care). Key recommendations from the York workshop were:

- establishment by the Department of Health of a nursing research advisory group
- mapping of current nursing research capacity
- development of innovative career paths
- establishment of research training fellowships and career scientist awards
- co-operation between funding councils
- pump-priming of potential centres of excellence
- recognition of the needs of nurses, midwives and health visitors in initiatives intended to promote the dissemination of research.

Many of these recommendations come from an appreciation of common deficits within health service R&D or from an acknowledgement of the need to address particular recognised capacity deficits in nursing, midwifery and health visiting.

The apparent overlap between the 1993 and 2000 strategy documents gives rise to a series of questions about how far the position of nursing with regard to R&D had changed in the intervening period. More specifically, the capacity-building efforts begun within the R&D programme itself may have helped to raise expectations but delivered little in tangible results beyond the language of hope and reassurance.

Building capacity

One might expect that the alleged commitment to building capacity within the R&D programme would have trained attention upon nursing and midwifery. But, despite the existence of the taskforce document (DoH, 1993), nursing, midwifery and health visiting receive little attention in an important research strategy document – *Research Capacity Strategy for the Department of Health and the NHS: A First Statement* (DoH, 1996). The relatively high proportion of discussion devoted to medical practitioners suggests that NHS R&D was seen primarily as medical, to be undertaken by doctors with the support of non-clinical researchers. Non-medical clinicians received almost no mention in the main body of the report even though the need for multidisciplinarity is acknowledged. The only substantial mention of nursing refers to the comparative lack of a research culture, and there is little appreciation of the potential contribution the profession could make. Non-medical health care professions do, however, merit a two-page annex which outlines the difficulties facing these disciplines in some detail, essentially covering ground similar to the 1993 Taskforce report. However, no recommendations were made as to how these difficulties might be addressed. More generally, no aspects of the strategy addressed the needs of nursing, midwifery and health visiting specifically. This is surprising given the report's recognition of the particular needs of the professions.

Notwithstanding the early consideration given to the issue of variable research capacity across the health professions and related disciplines (Lewis and Ritchie, 1995), this never led to the problem being the subject of sustained effective policy action. It was to be revisited after the 'First Statement' was published in

1996 (Workforce Capacity Development Group, 1998) indirectly through a Strategic Review Sub Group, set up under the chair of Professor Michael Clarke in 1999 (DoH, 1999b). Among its aims were to develop a strategy for the planning and review of spending in the NHS Research and Development Levy in accordance with the previous policy objectives; to examine opportunities and spending in areas of national priority; and to advise on the terms of reference and methods of working of expert groups reviewing these areas and other topics. One of the recommended areas for priority was the development of research capacity in terms of research training and career prospects (para. 7d). The group considered that a major weakness in the present R&D programme was the shortage of experienced health service researchers in well-developed career structures and that this shortage was a major threat to the R&D programme as a whole. It recommended that the NHS should focus capacity building on research skills vital to the NHS, which were in short supply (para. 27). The Group issued a report specific to the need for research in primary care, where 85 per cent of all health care problems in the NHS are managed (DoH, 1999b). The group identified a particular evidence gap in this sector, one characterised by the involvement of nurses and allied health professionals and their management of chronic conditions. This gap ranged across the whole range of research levels, from a 'basic science gap' to an 'implementation gap'. The incomplete nature of rehabilitation research was also highlighted in the Medical Research Council Topic Review of Primary Health Care (MRC, 1997), the King's Fund/Audit Commission Reports (Nocon and Baldwin, 1998; Sinclair and Dickinson, 1998) and a critical review of the evidence commissioned by the British Society of Rehabilitation Medicine (Turner-Stokes, 1999).

Notwithstanding the language used in the report, which refers to 'primary care' and 'general practice' interchangeably, it is unusual within government documents in that it makes numerous specific recommendations about the future R&D role and needs of nurses, midwives and health visitors. Thus the need to allow the small numbers of active non-medical clinical researchers in primary care to further develop their research roles is stressed, as is the necessity for support for successive generations of such researchers. Further recommendations note the need to influence statutory bodies responsible for the professions to permit or stipulate research expertise among those responsible for the preparation of clinicians of the future. These provisions are an important recognition of the needs and potential contribution of non-medical practitioners to the R&D agenda. However, what is lacking from the Mant report (DoH, 1997a) is a recognition of the extent of the need, the potential contribution and the required actions to address the former and facilitate the latter. Partly as a response to this perceived need a subgroup was set up. Having outlined some of the steps in capacity-building approaches that were beginning to emerge within the R&D programme, what then of other policy levers?

Research workforce

Given the size of the nursing, midwifery and health visiting workforce it might be expected that the role of these professions would make a strong showing in an examination of workforce needs for R&D within the NHS. *Developing Human Resources for Health Related R&D: Next Steps* (DoH, 1998a) goes further than *Research Capacity Strategy for the Department of Health and the NHS: A First Statement* (DoH, 1996) in recognising and specifying the particular difficulties faced by nurses and allied health professionals in addressing the R&D agenda. However, it is essentially limited, for although providing an excellent summary of these difficulties little is provided in the way of solutions. It is noteworthy that, having acknowledged the shortage of non-medical clinical researchers, no specific recommendation to remedy this situation is proposed, although the comments within the document with regard to integrated clinical and research careers may be particularly important in developing nursing and the allied health professions. Likewise, despite the size of this professional grouping, no recommendation in *Developing Human Resources* is targeted specifically at meeting the R&D needs either of this group as a whole or of nurse, midwives and health visitors in particular. This is perhaps unsurprising if the funding context for NHS R&D is examined (DoH, 1994a). It is entirely appropriate that no specific provision for one clinical discipline rather than another should be made. Moreover it is likely that a successful funding structure will be one that encourages the performance of the highest-quality research, and it is also likely that such research will be generated from an institution or discipline which has a strong research culture and track record. NHS research funding is designed, at least in part, to reflect these probabilities. The great problem with this approach is that it is by its nature conservative and in consequence neglects the opportunity costs which arise from failing to examine the potential within a profession to generate clinical practice which is effective and to investigate that practice. It is arguable that nursing, midwifery and health visiting have enormous potential of this kind which current funding arrangements and their workforce implications overlook. However, while it is welcome that a specific standard related to long-term capacity building will be required of bidders under the revised system, there is once again no discussion within the most recent R&D funding document of nursing, midwifery and health visiting and their particular needs, nor for that matter the capacity needs of the service as a whole (DoH, 2000a).

Making a difference

As mentioned above the York workshop (DoH, 2000a) took its impetus from the commitment expressed in Chapter 7 of *Making a Difference* (DoH, 1999a) to developing a strategy for nursing, midwifery and health visiting research. It is therefore potentially instructive to examine the role of R&D within this document. *Making a Difference* is apparently a cornerstone of government thinking with regard to the future preparation and role of nurses, midwives and health visitors. The document sets out how preparation for nursing, continuing education and a clinical career structure will change the potential contribution to be made by the professions to the health service. This contribution is seen as essential to modernising the NHS and improving the nation's health. However, although it has long been accepted that clinical practice and education for health care should be research based, research and development occupy little space within the report. Indeed, research activity does not receive a mention in the outline agenda for action presented in Chapter 2 of the document. It is instructive to examine the potential role for R&D in each key element of *Making a Difference*, and to compare this with the actual attention R&D receives within the document. It might be expected that Chapters 4, 5, 7, 8 and 10 (which deal with education and training, career frameworks, quality of care, leadership and working in new ways) would particularly call for a clearly articulated R&D component.

With regard to education and training, *Making a Difference* applauds the integration of nursing, midwifery and health visiting education into the universities but equally notes the perception that newly qualified nurses lack appropriate clinical skills. In this context the importance of teaching by those with recent clinical experience is emphasised. Unfortunately the opportunity to specify the relevance of clinical research to clinical skill, and therefore the need to ensure an adequate research infrastructure for the professions, is missed. We might reasonably expect that the clinical skill of those teaching learner nurses should be based on the most up-to-date evidence of clinical effectiveness. This evidence base has to come from somewhere, and ultimately this involves primary research into and carried out by the nursing, midwifery and health visiting professions. Thus it might be considered equally important for educators to be research active as to be clinically active, as in medical education (the yardstick used within the document for stating the importance of clinical activity among nursing, midwifery and health visiting educators). However, R&D is not mentioned in this chapter other than to note that interpretation and application skills relevant to R&D should be enhanced. This overlooks the need to create and support a context within which the material to be interpreted and applied can be created.

In Chapter 5 of *Making a Difference*, career frameworks are examined. Two major issues regarding career pathways in this document have particular implications for R&D: integration of research and clinical work, and the creation of the nursing, midwifery and health visiting consultant. With regard to the former the need for flexible career pathways and joint working between research and clinical work has been stressed in a number of documents, both with regard to the NHS generally (DoH, 1998a) and to specific areas of practice, including primary care (DoH, 1997a) and nursing, midwifery and health visiting (DoH,

1993). Unfortunately there is no recognition in *Making a Difference* that nursing, midwifery and health visiting might need to reflect the position in, for example, medicine, where movement between and integration of research and clinical roles is, however imperfectly, the norm. With regard to nurse consultantship the need is described for post-holders at this level to 'initiate and lead significant *practice, education and service* development' (italics added). Again, research is conspicuous by its absence, yet we might justifiably imagine both that research and research leadership would be considered essential components of consultantships (as in other disciplines) and that research skills would be essential to the effective realisation of practice, education and service development.

Within *Making a Difference* the strongest statement regarding R&D is made in the context of improving quality (Chapter 7) and the importance of a voice for nursing, midwifery and health visiting is identified. The importance of critical appraisal skills and research capacity building is explicitly stated (skills that are addressed later in this book – see Chapters 3 and 5 respectively). This is a welcome element of *Making a Difference*, and at this point in the document the relevance of R&D to career paths and consultantship is mentioned, as is the need to establish a cadre of individuals capable of securing an adequate evidence base for practice. However, nurse researchers might be forgiven for thinking that this single paragraph of intended activity is too insignificant within the document as a whole to permit confidence that a commitment to R&D is integral to *Making a Difference*.

In Chapter 8 of *Making a Difference*, while shortcomings of clinical leadership are noted, no mention is made of the great dearth within nursing, midwifery and health visiting of *research* leaders. Arguably such leadership must, on the one hand, be secured before appropriate R&D can be placed in the various other elements of *Making a Difference* and is a prerequisite of a strong R&D infrastructure within the professions. On the other hand, paradoxically, for leadership within nursing research to be a broad-based and sustainable activity, the well-recognised deficits in terms of preparation for research at every level within the professions must be addressed. (This is the topic of Chapter 6 of this book.) So much so that the importance of research and development for the health professions is recognised in the draft legislation for the Health Professions Council (DoH, 2001). For example, registrant or alternate members of the Council are expected to be 'wholly or mainly engaged in the practice, teaching or management of the profession, or in research into the profession for which he (*sic*) is registered and for which he seeks election' (p. 49). Good though intentions may have been they were never strong enough to sway the case for reform. The appointment of David Thompson as part-time Professor of Nursing Research within the DoH was to be welcomed but there were many other initiatives competing for policy makers' attention, not least that of quality, clinical governance and performance management.

Quality and clinical governance

Quality is said to be at the heart of the new NHS (DoH, 1998a), and we might expect that clinically excellent care would play a key role within clinical governance and that nurses, midwives and health visitors, by virtue of the sheer amount of care they deliver, would be key players in this forum. In order to occupy such key roles the professions arguably need not only a grasp of research appraisal (as outlined in *Making a Difference* among other documents) but also a series of strategies, activities and skills by which a continuing evidence base can be built. A number of documents are relevant to this issue. At a strategic level the processes by which clinical governance will be achieved are outlined in *A First Class Service* (DoH, 1998b), yet nursing, midwifery and health visiting receive little mention in the document. It is perhaps instructive that the 'duties of a doctor' are set out within the document as a highlight box but the duties of a nurse (midwife, health visitor, physiotherapist, psychologist, and so on) receive no mention. This lack of emphasis on professions other than medicine is of particular concern given the amount of contact and care provided by them.

Clinical governance is primarily concerned with standards and as a result, at least in the short term, with the dissemination of best evidence rather than the creation of new evidence. In consequence, there is little mention of R&D, even in those elements of the document concerning standard setting. For nursing, midwifery and health visiting this is problematic since the amount of care provided by these professions is great, but the evidence base behind it is at least as scanty as that for medicine. There is thus considerable potential for the professions to do harm to patients. In consequence it may be argued that there is a particularly pressing need for nursing, midwifery and health visiting to investigate their practice and create an evidence base in the future, yet there is no appreciation of this within the document. This is hardly surprising, given the generally low profile of the professions within it, but it is potentially a serious flaw, since we may end up with an immense area of care being provided not only without evidence but also, in the absence of a strategy to grow research within the professions delivering it, without a robust ability to construct that evidence in the future. Without such an ability it is doubtful how nursing, midwifery and health visiting can ever become evidence based, and one may construct at least two depressing scenarios: that care continues to be based upon current best evidence, which in many cases is at the level of clinical anecdote and 'expert testimony'; and that evidence for care is generated outside the profession, from disciplines with a more developed tradition in clinical research. Finally the need for nurses, midwives and health visitors to work in new ways is clearly laid out, and a number of potentially exciting new roles are identified, but scant reference is made to the need for adequate evaluation of such roles and no mention of either the need for robust research to underpin such evaluation or the potential for members of the nursing, midwifery and health visiting professions to undertake key roles in such evaluation and research.

Reform of R&D policy

As we can see, a growing case for reforming access to research resources was beginning to crystallise with greater clarity through many of the wider changes advocated within NHS health, nursing and R&D policy. Whatever the original motivation behind the drive for a strategic approach to NHS R&D at its inception ten years ago, it was becoming clear that health care research holds a central place in the present government's endeavour to establish performance management across the NHS. *The New NHS* (DoH, 1997b) sets out a policy priority of assessing the delivery of health care against new national standards and the reduction of unacceptable variations in performance (DoH, 1997b). Subsequent policy, both for the service as a whole and for R&D itself, has reinforced this aim. Among the many features of the Government's agenda has been the unprecedented weight given to evidence. Professional expertise alone is no longer sufficient guarantee of quality. Instead an elaborate apparatus of accountability and audit has grown up to scrutinise and rationalise professional decision making. New bodies, such as the National Institute for Clinical Excellence (NICE), aim to provide scientific guidance on current best practice regarding a range of specific issues. Though it is not the only body to produce them, NICE attempts to assemble the best research evidence in order to develop clinical guidelines for specific situations and treatments. Many such guidelines reflect NHS priorities and relate particularly to the National Service Frameworks (NSFs).

The intention of NSFs is that they set national standards and define service models for a specific service or care group, put in place programmes to support implementation and establish performance measures against which progress can be measured. Building on the frameworks for cancer and paediatric intensive care, the first two NSFs were for mental health (published in September 1999) and coronary heart disease (published in March 2000). At the time of writing there are six: coronary heart disease, mental health, older people, diabetes, children and renal disease. The NHS plans to produce one new topic a year. Each NSF has been developed with the assistance of an expert reference group that brings together health professionals, service users and carers, health service managers, partner agencies and others. In addition, each NSF includes a research agenda.

As part of a wider reform effort the present Government has sought to transform the funding and practice of the R&D funded within the NHS with the intention of increasing its quality, efficiency and relevance to the management of the service. In March 2000 a new development programme was set out (DoH, 2000a) which proposed a new structure for funding NHS R&D:

- NHS Priorities and Needs R&D Funding to support the development of the knowledge base required by the NHS
- NHS Support for Science to provide the NHS contribution to the science base which underpins or could underpin the service.

Aware of the implications for research capacity, the document also states that 'Where there is a shortage of the research skills needed to deliver these programmes, there will be specific initiatives to strengthen R&D capacity in particular disciplines, professions and service sectors' (para. 2.5).

In addition, a New Research Governance Framework, published on 1 March 2001, defines the broad principles of good research governance, sets standards, details the responsibilities of the key people involved in research, outlines the delivery systems and describes local and national monitoring systems. It also sets out arrangements to define and communicate clear quality standards delivery mechanisms to ensure that these standards are met and arrangements to monitor quality and assess adherence to standards nationally.

R&D and the professions

Throughout this period nursing and midwifery groups were actively endeavouring to influence funding agendas in a variety of ways, the most visible of which was through priority-setting exercises. In the most recent of these and drawing on the method of the original NHS R&D strategy the nursing, midwifery and health visiting professions developed their own priorities for research after an 18-month consultation process that involved over one hundred managers, clinicians and researchers (Kitson et al., 1997). Priorities were identified in care and caring practices, the health care environment, organisation and management, and the health care workforce. Many topics had a 'read-over' to health services research such as teamwork, informal carers, new technologies, the effectiveness of health alliances, workforce planning, continuity of care. Fourteen topics were submitted to the HTA (Health Technology Assessment) in 1998 although none were prioritised, but a number of themes (such as workforce, information technology and continuity of care) emerged for commissioning within the service delivery and organisation (SDO) arm of the R&D programme. The SDO's own themes were generated by a national listening exercise conducted with a wide range of lay, policy and professional constituencies. (Fulop and Allen, 2000). Follow-through work has been conducted to try to engage the research charity sector proactively in focusing upon research in nursing, midwifery and health visiting. Efforts have been made to influence the R&D funding agenda indirectly by identifying priorities that are relevant to that agenda and encouraging a focus on nursing, midwifery and health visiting questions and interventions.

The above professionally driven exercises came as close to defining demand as is possible: they tell us what the people working in practice want on the research agenda. It was therefore disappointing that the messages were not been taken up by funders. Significantly many priorities have a generic appeal and potential to impact on NHS services. Even if these exercises have not led directly to funding they have provided in some cases the opportunity to engage the support of the wider R&D community. This was one of the strengths of the RCN/Centre for Policy in Nursing Research exercise where funders and other stakeholders supported the initiative by agreeing to become members of the Strategic Alliance for Research in Nursing and Midwifery. Lack of resources meant the alliance remained a virtual entity. But significantly the difficulties that many groups have experienced in influencing priority-setting exercises had led the HTA to launch a consultative exercise led by Professor David Foxcroft, Oxford Brookes University, aimed at identifying ways of improving the participative process for agreeing the research agenda. Although opportunities presented themselves and pressure was applied these failed to shape up into strategic policy action.

Having mapped out some of the key policy drivers and developments within R&D, capacity building and policy related to nursing, there remains the significant sector of higher education (HE) which has exerted influence upon the case for investment. The addition of HE as an actor putting its policy weight behind the initiative helped solidify the case for change. Notwithstanding the position of nursing and midwifery, although improved overall within the RAE, this growth was reflected in grade inflation across the sector. Nursing and Midwifery's Unit of Assessment 10 was the lowest-ranked discipline in the league table of achievement.

Higher educational performance

This lowly position disguises a fact that is cause for much encouragement in terms of the growing capacity to do research within nursing and midwifery. Two of the authors of this chapter (AMR and MT) were involved in a recent study commissioned by the DH/HEFCE Taskgroup 3 to inform future policy on research within nursing, midwifery and allied health professions (AHP) (CPNR et al., 2001). The study was divided into two parts: a mapping study of research outputs and activity, and a policy justification study outlining the business case for investment. Significantly nursing, midwifery and AHP departments were generating increasing research income. The 50 departments responding to the survey showed an increase from £3m in 1996–97 to £9.7m in 1999–2000. The principal funders have been the Department of Health, NHS regional offices and trusts. HEFCE support for research has been £3m a year of QR (Quality Rating) funding to 11 departments in Unit of Assessment 10 (UOA), which covers nursing and midwifery. Some of the £7m a year which has gone to UOA 11 will have reached AHP departments, although we do not know the proportion. The capacity to do research has also been increasing: over the five-year period to 1998–99 nursing, midwifery and AHP research staff in universities have grown in number from 97 to 240; however, this represents only 3.9 per cent of the total staff of 6174. Comparable figures for other benchmark disciplines are from education with 7.6 per cent and social work/studies with 13.3 per cent.

In the RAE (Research Assessment Exercise) for 2001 the number of submissions in UOA 10 (which covers nursing, midwifery and health visiting) increased by 19 per cent – the second highest of any discipline. In addition the number of Category A and A* staff increased by 50 per cent over the 1996 figure – the second highest percentage of any discipline. However, the number of such staff, at 623, is still low in comparison with the total of full-time teaching staff. In UOA 11 (which includes the allied health professions) the submissions were 10 per cent higher than in 1996 but the number of academic staff increased dramatically by 57 per cent (the highest of any discipline) to 1066. However, we do not know what part of this increase can be attributed to the AHP disciplines. Postgraduate student numbers in nursing had also grown over the same time scale by 94 per cent and amounted to 3700 in 1998–99. All but 435 of these are part time. The bibliometric analysis we commissioned had shown a matching increase in published papers over the last ten years, although the outputs for nursing and midwifery have not increased since 1995.

Authors from hospitals and practice account for a substantial minority of the papers in all disciplines. In dietetics, midwifery, and speech and language therapy one in six of the papers had a foreign author (as a sign of international collaboration) and the same disciplines had a high number of authors from different addresses, indicating interuniversity collaboration within the UK. A high proportion of published papers revealed no funding source, implying they were self-funded: this percentage was 83 per cent for occupational therapy, 73 per cent for nursing, 71 per cent for physiotherapy, 57 per cent for midwifery, 46 per cent for speech and language therapy and 38 per cent for dietetics. In the NHS as a whole 47 per cent of funding of published papers is unacknowledged, which means largely unfunded. The UK government provides funding for the research behind 33 per cent of publications in all of biomedicine. Respondents to our questionnaire gave us information on their research outputs, which averaged out at only 1.8 papers over the whole of the last four years for the 1900 staff involved. They also told us the present number of PhDs among their staff, which was an average of 16 per cent of the total number. Finally the survey enquired about the number and type of collaborative links which nursing and AHP departments had with other departments or institutions. In nursing and midwifery it was usual to have two formal links with other disciplines and two with other institutions, but to have more than five collaborative arrangements with NHS-related organisations.

Demand for research

The demand for research is rarely identified or quantified so that in our research we decided to categorise it in three ways: policy- and R&D-driven demand, that identified by professional groups, and relative demand compared with other benchmarks. There was ample evidence of need but little of demand. Demand is a complex concept with both common-sense and technical meanings. For the purposes of the study we defined it broadly as the call for research to meet the needs and priorities of the NHS and to develop a secure and sustainable academic base for nursing, midwifery and AHPs within higher education. There is no simple way of measuring such demand and therefore we used indicators derived from a range of sources. For the purposes of the study we categorised demand in three ways, namely: professionally driven (that identified by the professional groups themselves); policy and R&D driven (that derived from the policy and R&D community); and relative demand (that is, measured against some reference point, benchmark or comparator). We dealt mainly with the first two categories: professionally driven, and policy and R&D community generated demand. The approach was pragmatic and relied upon the collection of data from existing sources and through rapid response consultation exercises. Indicators of demand could be found in a wide range of sources: recent health and R&D policy, the Health Technology Assessment (HTA) programme, Centre for Reviews and Dissemination (CRD), nursing and AHPs liaison with the National Institute of Clinical Excellence (NICE), two case studies of regional R&D funding patterns, and consultation with professional groups and practitioners.

The shortage of health service researchers is considered by some to be a threat to the NHS R&D programme as a whole and research in primary care in particular. A recent study referred to a vicious circle of disadvantage in which, because there were few well-qualified researchers (and little sustained investment in developing this capacity), the research outcomes were limited in number and quality. Three of the relevant professions (nursing, physiotherapy and occupational therapy) have recently carried out consultation exercises asking their members in which topic areas they thought research was a priority. These findings have been passed on to funders, but have had disappointingly little impact so far. A similarly wide range of opinions is collected by the panels of the Health Technology Assessment (HTA) Programme, whose role it is to prioritise topics for later NHS funding. We analysed a sample of the topics put forward and found that 10 per cent were potentially applicable to nursing, midwifery and AHPs. NICE has also been presented with a number of research topics to consider in the same disciplines. Our survey of demand involved an analysis of research proposals submitted to two NHS Regional Offices. This showed that a significant number by the relevant professions were not funded (although this may have been due to poor quality). Discussions with the Council of Deans of Nursing and the Research Forum of the Allied Health Professions served to confirm areas where they thought research was needed and there was demand for more research capacity and investment in young researchers.

We compared research activity in nursing, midwifery and AHPs with that in education and social work, two professional areas with similar profiles. In the case of education the weakness in research capacity and outputs was recognised in 1998 by the creation of a special teaching and learning research fund managed for HEFCE by the ESRC. This now has a budget approaching £23m which is used, among other things, to 'enhance the system-wide capacity for research-based practice in teaching and learning'. Social work as a discipline shares many of the same concerns as nursing, midwifery and the AHPs – no co-ordinating body for funding research, the need for an evidence base to inform practice – while it remains invisible as a discipline as far as many funders are concerned. Despite this its academic departments have succeeded in the RAE, with 16 per cent of departments gaining a rating of 5/5* (compared with 3 per cent in nursing and midwifery). A comparison of the 1998/99 research income of academic departments shows that nursing and AHP departments received the lowest proportions of QR and research council funding of all subjects.

Conclusion

There is good reason to be optimistic about research in nursing and midwifery. The policy mood has changed from strict multi-disciplinarity to one where it is considered politically accept-able to build capacity in targeted areas within health care. We welcome the research development awards for doctoral and post-doctoral fellows. PPP Foundation have invested significantly in separate fellowship scheme and partnership award schemes for doctoral and post-doctoral fellows, adding to research strength in nursing, midwifery and allied health professions. A new Nurs-ing, Midwifery Service, Delivery and Organisation programme within the NHS R&D Programme has been established and has embarked on a priority-setting exercise, commissioning from Spring 2003. But much more remains to be achieved. HEFCE have not yet declared the amount that they are prepared to invest in the joint scheme with the DoH, nor indeed what such funds may be used to support. There is an argument for trying to do something different and support research leadership or col-laboration in areas where the value-added will produce an identi-fiable pay-off. This may be at more senior levels or across the NHS and HE, not only in areas of priorities and needs. There needs to be provision for blue skies work and methodological development too.

Significantly too clinical governance is likely to feature more prominently as a lever of change. As reviews from the Com-mission for Health Improvement reveal, clinical effectiveness and research are often singled out for criticism as the source of disconnect between the evidence base required for clinical decision making (www.CHI.org). R&D will be expected to play an increasingly prominent role in quality improvement within the star-rated system. As the future unfolds those with influence need to constantly monitor the process and help to shape priorities, for example the great need to strengthen quantitative research capacity in nursing and to forge much better links with – and access to – the patient/user communities. Nursing has often claimed proximity to the patient as one of its defining charac-teristics. Its research repertoire must increasingly reflect that reality and turn sentiment into science if success it to be assured.

Key points

- Little is known of the impact of the nursing and midwifery workforce in the NHS.
- Stakeholder unity is needed to strengthen links with users of health care services.
- 'Payback' is needed to justify investment in R&D.
- Professional and policy drives are the catalysts for change.

References

CPNR (Centre for Policy in Nursing Research, R&D Forum Allied Health Professions, Association of Commonwealth Universities, CHEMS Consulting) (2001) *Promoting Research in Nursing, Midwifery, Health Visiting and Allied Health Professions.* Report to DH/HEFCE Taskgroup 3. Bristol: Higher Education Funding Council for England.

DoH (Department of Health) (1993) *Report of the Taskforce on the Strategy for Research in Nursing, Midwifery and Health Visiting.* London: Department of Health.

DoH (Department of Health) (1994a) *Supporting Research and Development in the NHS* (The Culyer Report). London: HMSO.

DoH (Department of Health) (1994b) *Working in partnership: Review of the Mental Health Nursing Review Team.* London: HMSO.

DoH (Department of Health) (1996) *Research Capacity Strategy for the Department of Health and the NHS: A First Statement.* London: HMSO.

DoH (Department of Health) (1997a) *R&D in Primary Care: National Working Group Report* (The Mant Report). London: Department of Health.

DoH (Department of Health) (1997b) *The New NHS: Modern, Dependable.* London: The Stationery Office.

DoH (Department of Health) (1998a) *Developing Human Resources for Health-related R&D: Next Steps* (The Pearson Report). London: Department of Health.

DoH (Department of Health) (1998b) *A First Class Service: Quality in the New NHS.* Leeds: Department of Health.

DoH (Department of Health) (1999a) *Making a Difference: Strengthening the nursing, midwifery and health visiting contribution to health and healthcare.* London: Department of Health.

DoH (Department of Health) (1999b) *Saving Lives: Our Healthier Nation*. London: Department of Health.

DoH (Department of Health) (2000a) *Research and Development for a First Class Service*. Leeds: Department of Health.

DoH (Department of Health) (2000b) *Towards a Strategy for Nursing Research and Development: Proposals for action*. London: Department of Health.

DoH (Department of Health) (2001) *A New Research Governance Framework*. http://www.doh.gov.uk/research/rd3/nhsrandd/research governance.htm (accessed 1 June 2002).

Fulop, N. and Allen, P. (2000) *National Listening Exercise: Report of the Findings*. NCCSDO, March.

HEFCE (Higher Education Funding Council for England) (2001) *Promoting research in nursing and the allied health professions*. Research report 01/64. London: HEFCE.

Kitson, A., McMahon, A., Rafferty, A.M. and Scott, L. (1997) On Developing an Agenda to Influence Policy in Health-Care Research for Effective Nursing: A Description of a National R&D Priority Setting Exercise. *NT Research*, 2(5): 323–34.

Lewis, J. and Ritchie, J. (1995) *Advancing research: Research workforce capacity in health and social care*. London: Social and Community Planning Research.

MRC (Medical Research Council) (1997) *Topic Review of Primary Health Care*. London: MRC.

Nocon, A. and Baldwin, S. (1998) Audit Commission for Local Authorities and the National Health Service in England and Wales. King Edward's Hospital Fund for London. *Trends in rehabilitation policy: a review of the literature*. London: King's Fund/Audit Commission.

Rafferty, A.M., Bond, S. and Traynor, M. (2000) Does Nursing, midwifery and health visiting need a research council? *NT Research*, 5: 325–35.

Sinclair, A.J., Dickinson, E.J. (1998) King Edward's Hospital Fund for London. Audit Commission for Local Authorities and the National Health Service in England and Wales. *Effective practice in rehabilitation: the evidence of systematic reviews*. London: Kings Fund.

Thompson, D. (2000) A Mapping Exercise of Current Nursing Research (January 1995–December 1999). Paper prepared for the Research and Development Division and Nursing Division of the Department of Health.

Turner-Stokes, L. (ed.) (1999) *Evidence for Effectiveness of Rehabilitation – A critical review*. London: Arnold.

Workforce Capacity Development Group (1998) *Developing Human Resources for Health-Related R&D: Next Steps*. London: NHS Executive.

3 International perspectives: collaborative conversations

Dawn Freshwater and Carol Picard

The aim of this chapter is to widen the focus of nursing research and to highlight that the organisation of nursing is heavily influenced by a number of international agendas and agreements. It is argued that nurses do not work in isolation in any country, and it is important for practitioners and researchers to locate themselves in the context of global developments. Established programmes of nursing research are now becoming more frequent with the growth of graduate programmes in nursing in many countries. As our knowledge base increases the validity of research evidence for use internationally requires an examination of applicability across borders. In the scholarship of discovery we must ask the question: is this knowledge valid for use with persons in other countries? The evidence of replicated studies may provide some answer to this question. Also, as the pool of nurse researchers in particular areas may be expanding unevenly, collaboration is a means of bringing together nurses with research interests in common to share talents and resources in addressing areas of common phenomena of concern.

Introduction

International research collaboration holds the promise of advancing nursing and health care knowledge. Nursing care is a global concern, and the movement of people across the national boundaries makes the understanding of health and nursing care problems important to examine internationally. The organization of nursing and health care within the UK is heavily influenced by a number of international agendas and agreements, often in negotiation with the World Health Organization (WHO) and members of the European Community. Within the wider context WHO sets the targets for health gain and health promotion; see for example the Alma Ata Declaration (WHO, 1978) which called for an acceptable level of health for all the people of the world by the year 2000. Complementing this strategy one of the International Council of Nurses (ICN) priorities for the 1988 to 1993 period was to work with national nurses' associations to encourage and facilitate the development of research in nursing and by nurses and the dissemination of research findings (ICN, 1987). From the perspective of over a decade we can see that the impact of nursing research internationally is growing but it is still far from gaining the recognition and uptake that skilled and knowledgeable professionals deserve and that the populations they serve need. All the more reason to gather strong professional resolve and unite in our drive to improve health care. In 1994 Oguisso (1994:198) wrote that reading nursing research reports and documents from all over the world convinced her that it was time for concrete actions such as vigorous fostering of nursing research. She cites the ICN – an international federation with, at that time, 106 member associations – as having a facilitative role in networking and dissemination. We would add that it is the enthusiasm of the individual that empowers such organizations. As Bishop (1994:146) remarked nearly a decade ago, and it still holds true:

> The harnessing of the potential within the nursing profession to make a major impact on the quality of health care is indeed a challenge. It is a challenge that has triggered many initiatives both large and small, research based and practice driven. Nursing research is not the prerogative of an elite few; it belongs to the profession and must be bedded into practice ... as we meet one challenge head on so another domes tumbling behind. What a blessing that we have such a large band of warriors, and how essential that we collaborate and strive together.

Common areas of interest: Finding one's colleagues

Looking to the literature

There are several ways to link nurse researchers across national borders. First is the extant literature, which gives a sense of the leaders in a respective field of research. The advantages to the literature sources are the accepted authority of peer-reviewed research findings. The challenge may be not finding all pertinent literature in languages other than English, particularly if abstracts are not written in English. Also, depending on the country, the nurse may not be able to access all sources cited in the literature since there may be those who publish in venues not accessible across borders. In many academic institutions faculty members have their own websites. Directly contacting experts in the field with your questions and areas of interest is often met with enthusiasm. Researchers want to see the reach of their work extended.

New technologies in the past decade have created the means for electronic communication. Access to knowledge sources and the electronic storage of research data can accelerate the research process itself. Through the use of e-mail, websites, listervs and other forms of technology the potential for linkages has expanded. Often access to such resources is through professional organizations as well as libraries.

International organizations and international conferences

Other ways to connect with nurse scholars are through organizations. Professional organizations with research in their mission, whether general, specialty specific or interdisciplinary, are natural ways to connect with researchers. For international linkages, seeking membership in organizations with international emphasis can put you in touch with research leaders. These organizations offer access to researchers through publications, conferences and other services. Conferences are an ideal forum for professionals to share examples of innovative and creative practice. There are an increasing number of conferences that focus on specialist areas of practice. The support for these groups and the subsequent dissemination of scholarly activities highlights the level of enthusiasm and commitment individual practitioners have to improving patient care. Often the number of attendees at specialist conferences is small, not least because of the increasing difficulties of releasing any great numbers of staff for professional development activities. However, those of you who have had the opportunity to share your work with like-minded peers at a conference will appreciate both the time, effort and reward that goes into articulating the complexities of professional practice.

International conferences have become a more frequent venue for the presentation of nursing research as the impetus for nursing knowledge becomes a global concern. The opportunity for dialogue at such conferences is a rich way to foster links for research. The benefit of the conference venue is the opportunity for discussion with other participants on their research interests as well on your ideas for future projects. The forging of relationships is essential to the success of an international research project since communication across time and space must be clear. Our conference experiences have been most positive in linking with nurse scholars in the United Kingdom, Canada and New Zealand. In some instances you might be looking for an expert researcher in a particular area and in other instances colleagues may be asking for your expertise and wanting to replicate a study or use a particular methodology in which you are versed.

Examples of international nursing organizations

Sigma Theta Tau International (STTI) and the International Association for Human Caring (IAHC) are two international organizations which hold conferences annually and use other means to link world scholars. Sigma Theta Tau International was founded in 1922 and is a global organization of over 150,000 active members. Its mission is to advance nursing knowledge worldwide. STTI is an international organization dedicated to creating a global community of nurses who lead using scholarship, knowledge and technology to improve the health of the world's people. This organization is an honour society with benefits to its members, but it also offers resources to all nurses worldwide. To support its mission STTI offers nurses worldwide access to products, at no cost, over the internet to support the connection of nursing researchers (www.nursingsociety.org). One product is The Registry of Nursing Research, which houses nursing research data, including the names of researchers who have registered along with information about their studies. Research variables and results are listed and nurses from around the world are invited to submit their work. The studies are entered by the researchers themselves, and nurses do not need to be STTI members to submit their research to the registry. Sigma

Theta Tau leaders want to make the registry a truly international tool by capturing all the extant nursing research conducted. They are inviting organizers of nursing research conferences to notify presenters of the opportunity to enter their work into this database. Right now the work of over 12,833 nurse researchers' works may be accessed through this service. Another STTI offering is the Literature Index, a free search tool where one can access research on concept areas of interest. This service indexes both nursing and interdisciplinary journals provided that 50 per cent or more of their articles are research based. This index includes publications from 1996 and is updated monthly. Another feature of the index is a link to Medline® abstracts. The society's journal, the *Journal of Nursing Scholarship*, is now available an online version by subscription or as a part of membership services. International authors are a part of most issues. Future plans for STTI's knowledge products will include online discussion listervs, a panel of experts and consultants, and products to get nursing knowledge to the point of care. Below is a diagram of the STTI resources.

One of the benefits of the international research conferences sponsored by STTI is the mix of experts and new researchers as well as clinicians who attend. For example, one of the authors recalls becoming interested in the research literature on hope and meeting Judith Fitgerald Miller, an authority in that area, at an STTI convention. A stimulating and spontaneous dialogue about her work ensued. Although the author decided not go in that direction with her own research, the dialogue was informative, encouraging and helped to reflect on the shape the work should take.

The International Association for Human Caring (IAHC) is committed to advancing the knowledge of caring and caring research within the discipline of nursing. It has as its five goals as an international organization to:

1. identify major philosophical, epistemological and professional dimensions of care and caring to advance the body of knowledge that constitutes nursing and to help other disciplines use care and caring knowledge in human relationships
2. explicate the nature, scope, and functions of care and caring and their relationship to nursing

3. identify the major components, processes and patterns of care and caring in relationship to nursing
4. stimulate and support nurse scholars worldwide to systematically investigate care and caring and to share findings with colleagues
5. share knowledge through publications and public forums.

Every year scholars and clinicians gather to present and discuss research on caring. The annual research conference has been held in Australia, Finland, Scotland and the United States, with plans for Canada in 2004. The 2003 conference in Boulder, Colorado used a model of presentation of research with an emphasis on dialogue with all participants. Nurses from 13 countries gathered last year for this association's conference in Boston, Massachusetts. Many of the research papers are later submitted to the organization's peer reviewed journal the *International Journal for Human Caring*, published three times a year. A listerv discussion group is available to members to continue the in-person dialogues. Professor Freshwater and US researcher on caring Dr Sherwood are its moderators. The website of the organization is www.humancaring.org.

Indeed, the authors of this chapter met at an IAHC conference in 1996 and realized they held common research interests in the use of the arts to foster reflective practice in nursing education. Through contact by e-mail and in person at IAHC conferences, and visits to each other's respective institutions, both decided to embark on a project funded by the NHS entitled 'Establishing consumer involvement: Innovative approaches to multidisciplinary education and health care provision', where consumers and students came together for dialogue and used the arts as a mode of expression. This partnership of researchers has led to other projects and linkages. For example, in 2000 Picard was in the UK to work on the above project and met with other nurse scholars at the University of Nottingham.

The International Council of Nursing (ICN) is another nursing organisation that attempts to bring together scholars from around the world. It states that it represents 'nursing worldwide, advancing the profession and influencing health policy' (http://www.icn.ch/abouticn). Representing nurses from more than one hundred and twenty countries, it is the world's first and widest-reaching international organisation for nurses, operated by nurses for nurses. It provides advice and support in the areas of professional nursing practice, nursing regulation and socio-economic welfare for nurses. It has three core goals:

- to bring nursing together worldwide
- to advance nurses and nursing worldwide
- to influence health policy

and five core values:

- visionary leadership
- inclusiveness
- flexibility
- partnership
- achievement.

The ICN has a very strong and compelling mission statement, one that aims to motivate and align efforts. Surely this is crucial if nursing is to develop a reputation for being a profession that has an international body of research knowledge that is both pragmatic and scientifically credible, whatever that might mean.

Academic and practice links for research

International post-doctoral fellowships are a way of linking with senior researchers in a particular area. In the age of electronic communication some fellowships do not always require extensive on-site time but can be structured to accommodate scholars at a distance. Most schools of nursing will list their post-doctoral opportunities on their websites.

Visiting professorships are another mode of establishing a connection with nurse researchers. In this case an established researcher travels to an institution for a specified period of time for collaboration. The benefit to fellowships and professorships is establishing ties that can be sustained once the visits are over. Partnerships between schools of nursing and clinical practice sites can make the most of such visiting scholars. For example, this spring Boston area institutions the MGH Institute of Health

Professions, Massachusetts General Hospital, Brigham and Women's Hospital and Spaulding Rehabilitation Hospital have collaborated to invite Neville Strump and Linda Evans, two eminent researchers in gerontological nursing, to present their work, lead clinical problem discussions and consult on research projects related to geriatric care. It is hoped that this convocation of educators, researchers and clinicians will lead to the development of research projects aimed at improving the care of elderly patients.

Linking academic and practice settings to foster clinical research has a new model with the Massachusetts General Hospital funding two PhD-prepared nurse researchers' salaries for a two-year period to enable them to seek major funding and to be released from their regular programme of work. These scholars have linkages to academic nursing programmes in Boston for additional support. This hospital has had nurse scholars from many countries visit and present their work and dialogue with clinicians and PhD-prepared staff. For example, in the past two years two groups of oncology nurse leaders from the United Kingdom came to Boston to the MGH Institute of Health Professions to meet with nurse scholars there and at the Massachusetts General Hospital and the Dana Farber Cancer Center for discussions on common areas of concern and potential for research collaboration. Similar opportunities exist in the UK and across other countries for new and experienced nurse researchers to develop collaborative networks in their specialist area. Memorandum of co-operation are being encouraged across an extensive number of international academic institutions and their practice links.

Listerv discussion groups are a convenient way to link scholars with similar interests and are becoming common in other nursing organizations. The Royal Windsor Society for Nursing Research (research-nurses@canada.com) is an example of a listerv with a global membership. Other examples are the nurse scholar groups whose work is based on the nursing theory of Parse and Newman, (Parse, 1987; Newman, 1994). The International Council of Nurses Research Workgroup and the WHO Collaborating Centers for Nursing and Midwifery target research problems identified as international concerns by their parent organizations.

The need for clarity in purpose, processes and intended outcomes

Once you are linked to international colleagues the logistics of conducting international research must be addressed. First there must be a clarity of purpose: what do we wish to accomplish? Are all researchers clear on the purpose of the project? A strategy to ensure this is to engage in a dialectic with the project team, thus enabling everyone to have the opportunity to give their understanding of the project goals. Having addressed and identified the clarity of purpose it is also important to identify the process by which the research team will dialogue and share ideas. Clarity of intended outcome requires the collaborators to focus on how findings will be shared, the need for written agreements such as the memorandum of co-operation should be discussed. It is also worthwhile debating and agreeing such sensitive issues as intellectual property rights, copyright and ownership. This is of particular importance when thinking around publications of papers and reports.

Issues of the ethical conduct of the study will be influenced by research ethics committees approval variations from country to country and institution to institution. In other situations, persons involved in such studies must submit credentials to the host institution for approval as a researcher. Of course, even though many countries speak and use English there is still a need to examine research and ethics tools for language and cultural sensitivity.

Travel scholarships

As we have highlighted, there are numerous benefits from working in partnership with international colleagues. One way of enjoying an in-depth and 'close up' encounter with colleagues in other countries is through travel scholarships. There are a number of such scholarships that are available for both nurses and other health care professionals. However, there are also some that focus solely on the development and improvement of patient care through nursing practice. One such organisation is the Florence Nightingale Foundation. The Florence Nightingale Foundation offers travel scholarships to all nurses, midwives and health visitors who are registered with the Nursing and

Midwifery Council (NMC) and who are working within the UK. Scholarships are awarded for 'projects connected with the applicant's field of work and which will benefit their patients/ clients and the professions more widely' (http://www.florence-nightingale-foundation.org.uk).

Two other travel awards that we will mention here, although of course there are many more that we cannot refer too, are the Harkness Fellowships and the Fulbright Scholarships. Harkness Fellowships enable professionals with substantial experience in their own field of practice to spend up to one year in the USA. The Harkness programme encourages professional leaders to benefit from new ideas, practices and contacts in the USA with a view to 'enhancing UK developments: to build enduring relationships of value to professional communities on both sides of the Atlantic: and to sustain an international network of experts and practitioners addressing major social policy issues in a practice way'. The Fulbright programme, established in 1946, is the world's largest bi-national education programme. It operates in over 140 countries, administering a range of awards for professionals wanting to study in other countries (http://www.fulbright.org).

Key points

- Collaboration across countries is key to professional growth.
- There is great value in accessing individuals from other nations who share your professional interests.
- Professional organizations are only as good as the enthusiasm of their membership.
- Opportunities exist for travel to develop professional expertise.

References

Bishop, V. (1994) Prevention and Primary Health Care Delivery Challenges. In Fitzpatrick, J.J., Stevenson, J.S. and Polis, N.S. (eds) *Nursing Research and its Utilization*. New York: Springer.

ICN (International Council of Nurses) (1987) Blueprint for ICN Programme 1988–93 toward more effective participation in Health Policy Making and Health Care Delivery, approved by the CNR at its 1987 meeting, Auckland, New Zealand.

Newman, M. (1994) *Health as expanding consciousness.* New York: National League for Nursing Press.

Oguisso, T. (1994) Nursing Research Training and Career Development Around the World. In Fitzpatrick, J.J., Stevenson, J.S. and Polis, N.S. (eds) *Nursing Research and its utilization.* New York: Springer.

Parse, R.R. (2001) The human becoming school of thought. In Parker, M. (ed.) *Nursing theories and nursing practice.* Philadelphia: F.A. Davis.

World Health Organisation (WHO) (1978) Alma Ata Declaration, WHO.

4 The appreciation and critique of research findings: Skills development

Dawn Freshwater

As has been indicated in previous chapters developing a research-wise culture must be a part of any health care professional's ethos and indeed the ethos of a National Health Service (NHS) that is embracing a modernisation agenda. This requires a number of skills, some of which are addressed in this book. This chapter aims to help the reader to feel confident when faced with assessing and evaluating research, whether this is via formal papers, at conferences, in the clinical setting or in the classroom. In order to effect this aim it is necessary to undertake a brief survey of contemporary developments such as evidence-based practice and also to indicate the historical progression of methodological discourse in nursing research. This chapter is not, however, an outline of the relative merits and shortcomings of the various research paradigms and methods; there are a plethora of texts available to assist the practitioner in understanding these philosophical differences. Rather, as the title suggests, it aims to focus on the processes of evaluating and critiquing research.

Introduction

The need for organisations to provide effective, quality health care has been the subject of a number of policy and strategy documents within both the NHS and independent sectors of health care. Clinical governance is seen as one strategy that will enable employers to subject their organisation to scrutiny and to develop a competent workforce that meets customer and organisational needs.

For clinical governance to be effective, that is, to deliver improving standards of patient care in primary care groups, health authorities and acute trusts, new skills will be required throughout these organisations, These include effective leadership, clinical audit, and quality monitoring and improvement, as well as a wide range of education and professional development initiatives that monitor and develop the competence of the workforce. In addition, as outlined in earlier chapters, in order to meet these and other emerging agendas such as the requirement for continuing professional development and the drive towards evidence-based practice, nurses are increasingly expected to have the skills to appreciate and critically evaluate the growing body of evidence available to support best practice.

It is widely accepted then that a skilled and knowledgeable workforce is essential in order to achieve many of the strategic objectives highlighted by a variety of policy documents and reports, including the NHS Plan (DoH, 2000) and the National Service Frameworks, that are emerging for specific areas of care, including cancer care, diabetes, elderly care and mental health. Education and training for health care professionals has to take account of these and future policy changes if they wish to produce the competent and relevantly educated practitioners of the future. It is essential that the products of faculties and departments in higher education are viewed as fit for purpose while also being perceived as providing value for money. However, what is not always acknowledged is the need for the workforce to be competent in the appreciation, understanding and critique of research methods, their findings and their utilisation in practice: skills that are essential to the successful professional development of the individual and the implementation of any policy initiative.

The implications for higher education in developing and sustaining a research-competent workforce with the capacity to deliver, develop and generate policy and knowledge for quality nursing practice will be addressed in detail in Chapter 6. This chapter deals specifically with the skills of understanding and critiquing research, the methods used and the implications of how the findings are disseminated. Before moving into this area I will spend sometime outlining the significance of the recent drive towards evidence-based practice and its influence on the choice of approaches to research.

Evidence-based practice

The term evidence-based practice has become a well-rehearsed mantra of health care professionals over the past decade. For some it is a *bête noire* (Risdale, 1996), while for others it is undoubtedly the new, very welcome fashion. A definition of evidence-based medicine was provided in Chapter 2, where it was posited that nursing research, and as such evidence for effective clinical nursing practice, have traditionally been developed within the dominant paradigm of technical rationality. In contemporary society perhaps the most privileged form of knowing in the world is through science. It is so embedded in the implicit belief structure of our thinking that scientific proof has become equivalent to truth. Its influence, resources and epistemological dominance in government, the academy, industry, commerce and of course nursing and health care is highly visible (Freshwater, 2000; Neville, 1989). Empirical ways of knowing have been held in high esteem and have been dominant in health disciplines. While nursing is not simply about conscious and rational processes (witness the plethora of literature on the subject of tacit, intuitive and reflective experiential knowledge (see Rolfe, Freshwater and Jasper (2001); Rolfe (1998, 1996); Johns and Freshwater (1998)) for an in-depth examination of these issues) it has had to operate in a world in which scientific methods of understanding predominate and in which the legitimacy for practice increasingly rests upon the principles of science.

Recent paradigm shifts in ways of understanding and explicating human experience mean that more fitting approaches to understanding and representing knowledge have come to be accepted within the scientific community. In what has been called the postmodern world, the certainties of a bedrock of scientific truth which exists in codifiable and system form have been subject to sharp scrutiny (Lyotard, 1984). In the realms of philosophy and social theory, postmodernism has encouraged the realisation that not only are there many ways of knowing and understanding the world but also that the privileged position of particular forms of scientific discourse may be misplaced. As Polanyi (1962) has argued, this tacit knowledge can be explored but not by the classic means of making explicit through reductive analysis.

Different approaches to research

Beliefs about the 'correct' way of researching the social world has led to numerous discussions and debates regarding the relative merits and limitations of quantitative and qualitative approaches to research. Indeed, as Blaxter, Hughes and Tight (2001) note, the debate has at times resembled 'a veritable war zone' (p. 60). The quantitative and qualitative paradigms do offer a basic framework for dividing up knowledge into separate camps, yet even within these camps there are debates about what forms of knowledge and evidence are seen to be valid. While this debate continues new approaches to research have been developed and are being refined, these include postmodern and post-structuralist approaches, interpretative and critical reflexivity, constructivist and narrative methods. For the new student, learning about research and evidence can be a minefield, let alone questioning and evaluating how specific research findings relate to professional practice.

Moran (1998) uses a tripartite ontology based on Greek thought to differentiate distinct forms of research into Mysterious, Intelligible and Sensible. Much of nursing falls between the Mysterious and Sensible, between the unfathomable/unspeakable and that of the practical ground of our senses, and should thus be considered as belonging to the middle domain of the Intelligible. Moran says that the Intelligible is affected by both: 'it is inspired by the Mysterious and confronted by the Sensible' (Moran, 1998:123) He stresses that while the Intelligible connects and interfaces the other two domains it has its own order of knowledge and understanding. The analogy is that of H_2O which exists in three distinct states: ice, water and steam. Although the liquid state of water lies between the other two, it has its own distinct properties.

Moran suggests that quantitative research is appropriate when applied to the Sensible where outcomes can be clearly measured and the parameters of the research well controlled. This does not apply to all of nursing which deals with questions of meaning arising from the subject's interior world. He suggests that qualitative research is more suited to the exploration of phenomena that cannot be easily reduced to external behaviours without absurdity.

Whereas Moran makes the case for defining the Intelligible in terms of relationality and dialogue as necessary to enable an interior reality to reveal itself, a simpler way to make the distinction is between open and closed systems. The classical scientific method operates best within a closed system in which the parameters of the research can be tightly controlled and the criteria of generalisability, reliability and validity can be applied. I would suggest that the actual process of nursing is a paradigm example of an open system as it is open (and indeed recent policy initiatives demand this openness) to feedback and new information being exchanged. If some nursing theories have become somewhat closed this reflects more on the politics of the culture than on the nature of nursing practice.

The problem in qualitative research that has spent many years attempting to meet the standards of the traditional scientific forum, namely, generalisability, reliability and validity, is that the researcher is considered to be outside the frame. Attempts are made to eliminate any bias and to make the questioning process as neutral possible. This means that the while the researcher is open to feedback in terms of the design of the question he or she is attempting to eliminate his or her subjective response.

Objectivity and subjectivity

New ideas from Braud (1998), Rowan (1998), Freshwater and Rolfe (2001) and Alvesson and Skoldberg (2000) on transformational research offer a step beyond qualitative research in recognising the impossibility of the neutrality of the questionnaire/researcher and, rather than trying to cancel out bias, take this as an interesting element in the research process. Rather than simply acknowledging the impact of the researcher and trying through intersubjective means to minimise it, transformational research requires subjective reflexivity as necessary for exploring the subtle meaning of complex human experience. It requires a paradigm shift away from objectivity, not so much to intersubjectivity but to ideas of authenticity and interdependence. In nursing, for example, the material does not arise solely from the patient but comes through the collaboration of nurse and patient (see Freshwater, 2002 for clinical examples of this type of research). In this new perspective research is seen as an inter-dependent process that relies heavily on dynamic communication between researchers and practitioners. In transformational research the researcher lives through the experience of the patient rather than gaining knowledge about the patient experience.

Scientist–practitioner

Evidence based on the analysis of nursing outcomes (see Roth and Fonagy, 1996; McLeod, 2001; Hemmings, 1999) is some-times referred to as the scientist–practitioner approach and arises out of practices and procedures in such allied professions as psychology and medicine. It is often the case that publicly funded and market-orientated therapy systems such as public services have to provide some evidence of efficacy using this methodology (Rose, 2000; Corney, 1999).

Evidence based on the analysis of the process of therapeutic interventions (Hill and Corbet, 1993) – for instance, the work of Carl Rogers at Ohio State University in the 1940s and at the University of Chicago in the 1950s – involves the detailed analy-sis of professional–patient interactions with a view to identifying the therapeutic attitude and interventions which are therapeuti-cally efficacious. Rogers's work included the design of measures to evaluate the nature of the client response to practitioner attitudes and interventions. Again this type of research falls foul of the social context within which research operates, with the research often being undertaken by trained researchers and not necessarily by practitioners themselves, adopting similar practices to those of psychology.

Practitioner–researcher

Evidence based on the reflexive analysis of clinical experience, which is sometimes referred to as the practitioner–researcher approach, addresses the research–practice gap. This is relevant to current public debates about health care since some commenta-tors have argued that problems have arisen because academically trained health professionals have not been able to integrate their knowledge with everyday practice. It arises out of the practice of nursing itself, is thus familiar to the vast majority of practitioners, and can only be undertaken by practitioners. Historically it is the largest single type of writing in the profession and forms the central methodology on the majority of nursing courses.

This chapter does not seek to explore the emphasis of this and the scientist–practitioner perspectives in great depth. For further and more detailed analysis the reader is directed to the references at the end of the chapter. However, it is worth noting that there are substantial differences in the way in which professional practice is viewed by the scientist–practitioner approach and practitioner–researcher approach. These can be summarised as follows:

- The scientist–practitioner looks for explanatory, predictive theories; the objective of the practitioner–researcher is problem solving.

- The scientist–practitioner attempts to arrive at general statements about a large area of reality; practitioner–researchers attempt to arrive at concrete statements about local and contingent situations.

- The scientist–practitioner tends to take the line of impersonal objectivity, minimising bias; the practitioner researcher develops professional insights and findings based on a combination of knowledge, experience and empathic understanding.

Motivation for research

The particular approach/perspective that an individual takes when engaging in the research process will be dependent upon his or her rationale for conducting the research. It is important that the professional spends sometime reflecting upon his or her motivations for the research whatever paradigm they align themselves with. Indeed it is crucial that the question and the motivation for research determine the methodological approach, rather than the method dictating the shape and nature of the question. The professional needs to reflect on the situation and the actions he or she is taking, with the motives for certain choices being justified and verified.

William Braud (1998) argues that there are three main motivations for conducting research; to:

1. learn as much as we can about others, the world and ourselves in order to predict and control
2. understand the world in the service of curiosity and wonder
3. learn to appreciate the world and delight in its bountiful nature.

The first motivation might be related to the scientist–researcher model. Braud (1998) argues that this particular motivation serves security and adaptation and, I would add, brings in an important utilitarian dimension to research. He suggests that 'The search for universal laws – a nomothetic approach – is quite consistent with these motivations; knowledge of prinicples of great generality increases the ability to predict and control' (p. 53). The methods that support this type of research are usually experimental and quasi-experimental designs.

The second two motivations have much in common with the practitioner–researcher model: 'There is an interest in discovering nature's themes and variations' (p. 54). The focus here is on the concept of discovery and the wonder that accompanies discovery with the unpredicatability and unexpectedness of professional practice being as valued as the predictable and the expected. Thus a satisfying research outcome might be 'the presentation of a detailed map of some new territory or the revelation of some previously unknown trails and pathways in an old territory (Braud, 1998:54).

Whatever the motivation for the research, it is crucial that the professional begins with a question of great interest and importance to them, an area of enquiry that is driven from a heart-felt desire. This will affect not only the enthusiasm of the investigator and therein the successful completion of the project but also the meaning and learning derived from the experience. I move on now to the importance of the literature in supporting the investigation and investigator in their endeavour. Whilst the literature might be apportioned differing levels of significance across different methodological approaches, it is nevertheless of importance to all research at some point in the enquiry.

The literature review

A research study usually, although not always, starts off with a problem or question. Whatever the stimulus the research question is not always immediately suitable for focused research, requiring some exploration of its theoretical frame of reference. The development of a research question is addressed in more detail in Chapter 5. What I am concerned with here is the role of the literature in shaping the frame of reference for the study. It is also important to observe the distinction between research literature, conceptual or theoretical literature, and other forms of literature such as works of fiction, biography and poetry.

Reading research papers

Any nurse conducting a research project will almost invariably find him- or herself involved in a significant amount of reading, although as already mentioned the nature and timing of this reading will largely depend upon the chosen research method. Blaxter, Hughes and Tight (2001) argue strongly for the importance of reading when carrying out research, identifying ten reasons for doing so; to:

1. gain ideas
2. ascertain what other researchers have done in a similar field
3. expand perspectives and contextualise research questions
4. enhance direct personal experience
5. lend some weight to developing arguments
6. help clarify one's own position and maybe stimulate a change of opinion
7. effectively criticise what others have done
8. have the opportunity to learn more about research methods and their application to practice
9. identify gaps in research

and because

10. writers need readers!

It is interesting to note that the motivation for reading embedded within this list appears to be mostly extrinsic. Many practitioners and researchers read because they feel stimulated to do so from some intrinsic motivating factor. Indeed the motivation for research itself is usually based largely in intrinsic motivation, although this is almost always in the context of the individual's clinical practice. This is an important point, because the motivation for conducting a particular piece of research links directly to the amount of reading that is carried out and indeed what sort of reading is done.

Knoll Hoskins (1998) notes that the nature and purpose of the intended study directs the primary purpose of the literature review. She suggests that a study designed using quantitative methodologies will use the literature as an orientation to what is already known, to provide a conceptual or theoretical framework and to gain an indication of the appropriate research design, instruments and measurements. Whilst the conduction of a literature review prior to the data collection is controversial in qualitative studies, a preliminary review of the literature may be carried out for a variety of reasons. It can open the researcher to the complex nature of the phenomena under investigation, including the context and culture of the phenomena. It can also signify how the study might contribute to extant knowledge.

Typically sources of literature fall into two categories: primary sources or those written by the investigator, and secondary sources, those prepared by someone other than the original researcher. Whilst it is important to read as many different sources or texts as possible so as to encounter a range of views and forms of presentation, journal papers are often considered the prime source of information for keeping up to date. There are several reasons why the literature warrants this key 'prime source' status.

1. Refereed announcements of new research findings relevant to health professionals appear in the first instance in the literature aimed at health professionals.
2. Journal papers that report studies in their primary source normally provide sufficient detail of both methods and results for the reader to assess the relevance of the findings and, importantly, their application to the practitioner's own clinical environment.

3. The literature available for health professionals is indexed fairly extensively and is available electronically (and increasingly in full text form). There is little doubt that technology has facilitated the timely location of research papers and has of late become a useful source of secondary reviews and syntheses. It is important therefore that the investigator evaluate the perspective offered in the secondary source before accepting it uncritically.

As I have already indicated research papers are just one form of literature to be explored. However, the verification of research findings as described by the scientist–practitioner community usually takes place at the point of publication, with assessment for publication acting as the measure of the scientific quality of the research. This is to say that peer review for publication in a scientific journal acts as one form of critical appraisal. Scientific journals make high demands on their authors and often do not publish papers when the methodology was less convincing or did not follow a traditional format. This obviously has implications for the publication of practitioner–researcher based research which is often rejected by the more renowned international journals. It is important therefore to search the full range of literature sources to arrive at a fuller picture of the phenomena under consideration. In addition to exploring a full range of sources, including for example books, reports, letters and diaries, documents from meetings, the popular media and computer-generated materials, it is also worth bearing in mind other distinguishing factors. Within these and other sources reading material falls into a number of categories, which Blaxter, Hughes and Tight (2001) describe as:

- published and unpublished
- contemporary and classic works
- introductory and overview texts
- edited collections and literature reviews
- methodological and confessional writings.

Critical appraisal can and does of course take place in other arenas. Conferences, seminars and workshops can all support the constructive criticism and enhance the quality of research.

Academic institutions also act as critical verifiers of completed and ongoing research studies. The remainder of this chapter will focus on the skills of critical appraisal; however it is worth pointing out here the importance of organising your reading in order to maximise the efficacy of the time you have available.

Organising your reading

Because new information regarding nursing practice, research and education usually appears first in the peer-reviewed nursing journals it makes sense to devote part of one's time to pursuing that literature. Depending on your clinical field there are many specialist update services as well, however these derivatives often only appear after the original journal publication and are frequently based on unstated selection policies. Clearly you will need to develop an aggressive strategy to manage the wealth of literature available.

- Restrict your regular reading to mainly peer-reviewed journals that provide the best yield of papers for your own areas of clinical interest.
- Scan the methods and results of these papers to determine whether they are likely to be of direct importance for your own clinical practice.
- Ensure a diversity of literature drawing upon primary, secondary and other less obvious sources.
- Having discovered papers of potential interest scan the titles and note whether or not the paper is an original paper, a critical review, a meta-analysis or so on. At this stage check out whether or not the paper is of direct relevance to your research study/ clinical practice. If it is then examine the paper in further detail to assess if the basic methods are sound before going on to appraise the paper in detail.

Developing the skills of critical appraisal

The importance of critical appraisal skills have been outlined by the Department of Health in *Making a Difference* (DoH, 1999).

It could be argued that a researcher needs to carry out research in order to be able to read research critically, and there is no doubt that the experience of carrying out research gives one more insight into the research process. However, as Stevens et al. (1993) argue, it is possible to evaluate research with no previous experience.

There is no great mystery to the ability to read research critically. While it does require some knowledge, it is above all else a skill. As such the more you practice it the better you become, just as you would if you were learning to play a musical instrument or to drive a car. Herein lies a concern, in that like any other skill that is learned, once the skills of critical appraisal are learnt you can easily get into bad habits and taking short cuts. From a research perspective being critical pertains to the justified and considered examination of what other authors or speakers have said regarding the subject under investigation. During this process the researcher learns to entertain several contradictory ideas simultaneously while concurrently comparing and contrasting these ideas with their own opinions. Developing the skills of critical reading feeds directly into the development of writing critically and analytically and as such is fundamental to the evolution of a research portfolio through publication and presentations and, of course, reflection on/in practice (Rolfe, Freshwater and Jasper, 2001).

A critical reading of the literature, then, goes beyond a mere description of what has been read to include a personal response. Moreover the personal response not only relates different writings to each other but also offers alternative positions and vantage points. Critical appraisal of research is not just about identifying negative aspects of the literature under scrutiny; there are strengths and weaknesses in every paper which need to be assessed and addressed in a balanced way. When reading a paper it is useful to divide your initial analysis into two components, the first focusing on the literary product itself (that is, the wrapping), the second on the content (what is inside the wrapping). Learning to be critical of what you are reading helps you to assess the logic and rationale of arguments and ask questions that go beyond the text and what it is saying (Peelo, 1994). I would argue that in order to undertake a full critical appraisal the reader must also reflect on how he or she is interacting with the writing. In other words in what way is the writing stimulating the reader, how does it resonate with the reader's personal experience and to what extent is the reader rewriting him- or herself and his or her practice in relation to the text. Most research texts offer a framework for critical evaluation of research findings. What follows is a basic guide to the journey through the stages of the research process, highlighting the areas which affect the credibility of the study.

When analysing the contents of the material in more detail the process is made easier if the paper is broken down into smaller sections or substructures. Where these subsections are less obvious the reader can use the basic structure of introduction (abstract), methods, results and discussion to guide his or her analysis.

Introduction

You will need to ask to what extent are the questions or aims posed in the introduction relevant to the topic that you are investigating. Once this has been determined it is worthwhile at this early point to decide if the questions have already been answered adequately elsewhere and, if so, what can be gained from reading the paper in hand. You should also be able to get a sense of the context within which the research was undertaken which may help you to decide whether or not you wish to continue with the reading. Having decided that the paper is relevant and of sufficient interest to pursue you might like to assess the literature review or the background against which the researchers have posed their question/aims.

Methods

Whilst this chapter is not focusing on methodology, it is important to emphasise the importance of understanding research approaches and differing methods of applying research theories and philosophies. When reading a paper for methods you will need to ask to what extent the design of the study is appropriate for best answering the questions posed earlier. Other questions that might be considered include those related to the instruments, the sample and to the intervention. For example, how clear is the connection between ideas or concepts and the instruments used?; is the population and the population sample defined?; was the sample size appropriate to the method and the question being posed?

Results and analysis

Results of research studies will obviously vary enormously in their representation, not least because of the variety of research methods available. Whether the findings being evaluated originate from within the quantitative, qualitative or new paradigm research there are some basic questions that can be asked when reading the findings for credibility. Are the outcomes of the research sufficiently described in order that you can assess their clinical importance? Are the results presented in an easily understandable way, including the use of figures, tables and illustrations? Where relevant, was the response rate satisfactory?

Discussion

The discussion is often the point at which the writer demonstrates an awareness of the methodological limitations of the study. It is also the opportunity to acknowledge any difficulties encountered in conducting the study. All research is fraught with difficulties; however, if they are identified and described, the reader may have more confidence in the results themselves. Important questions to ask of the work at this stage include, are the conclusions drawn justified by the data presented?; are the findings compared and contrasted with other published research, both supportive and conflicting?

Researchers often make assumptions about the knowledge and understanding of the target audience, using all sorts of jargons and terms. As already indicated when critiquing a paper it is just as important to be aware of the 'wrappings', that is, the literary product itself. Has the author justified the use of his or her terms? It is a common error on the part of the reader to assume what the investigator means where the meaning is not made explicit. In other words, the reader makes assumptions about assumptions! A final point on the wrapping of the paper: investigators are often so deeply embedded in their subject matter that they may omit certain relevant information. Thus one must learn to read between the lines and identify what may have been accidentally, or indeed deliberately, omitted.

Conclusion

Evaluating research is the business of every health professional, even those who do not consider themselves involved in research. Quality care hinges on the understanding, implementation and development of research. The implementation of findings from sources other than your own area of practice must be undertaken with caution and only after critical appraisal. However, any practitioner interested and motivated to bring about change within his or her own practice should also do so in a responsible and accountable manner, critically appraising his or her own findings and of course disseminating them to the wider audience for further critique.

Key points

- Creating an environment conducive to learning is critical to the success of any research programme.
- Development of a strategy to manage available literature should be established early on.
- Conferences, seminars and workshops provide a space for critical appraisal of ongoing work.
- The process of nursing is an example of an open system of research.

References

Alvesson, M. and Skoldberg, K. (2000) *Reflexive Methodology*. London: Sage.

Blaxter, L., Hughes, C. and Tight, M. (2001) *How to Research*. 2nd edn, Buckingham: Open University Press.

Braud, W. (1998) Integral Inquiry: Complementary ways of knowing, being, and expression. In Braud, W. and Anderson, R. (eds) *Transpersonal Research Methods for the Social Sciences*. London: Sage.

Corney, R. (1999) Evaluating clinical counselling in primary care and the future. In Lees, J. (ed.) *Clinical counselling in primary care*. London: Routledge.

DoH (Department of Health) (2000) *The NHS Plan*. London: The Stationary Office.

Freshwater, D. (2000) *Transformatory Learning in Nurse Education*. Portsmouth: Nursing Praxis International.

Freshwater, D. (ed.) (2002) *Therapeutic Nursing*. London: Sage.

Freshwater, D. and Rolfe, G. (2001) Critical Reflexivity: A politically and ethically engaged research method for nursing. *NTResearch*, **6**(1): 526–37.

Hemmins, A. (1999) Assessment of psychological change and the future of practice of clinical counselling. In Lees, J. (ed.) *Clinical counselling in context*. London: Routledge.

Hills, C.E. and Corbett, M.M. (1993) A perspective on the history of process and outcome research in counselling psychology. *Journal of counselling psychology*, **40**(1): 3–24.

Johns, C. and Freshwater, D. (1998) *Transforming Nursing through Reflective Practice*. Oxford: Blackwell Science.

Knoll Hoskins, C. (1998) *Developing Research in Nursing and Health*. New York: Springer.

Lyotard, J.F. (1984) *The post modern condition. A report on knowledge*. Manchester: Manchester University Press.

McLeod, J. (2001) *Practitioner Research in Counselling*. London: Sage.

Moran, T. (1998) *Aging and Mental Health*. HCRA Research Training Institute and Washington, DC: Mental Health Policy Resource Center.

Neville, B. (1989) *Educating Psyche*. Victoria, Australia: Collins Drove.

Peelo, M. (1994) *Helping students with study problem*. Buckingham: Open University Press.

Polanyi, M. (1962) *Personal Knowledge: Towards a post-critical philosophy*. London: Routledge and Kegan Paul.

Risdale, L. (1996) *Evidence Based Practice. A critical reader*. London: W.B. Saunders.

Rolfe, G. (1996) *Closing the theory practice gap – a new paradigm for nursing*. Oxford: Butterworth Heinemann.

Rolfe, G. (1998) *Understanding and researching your own practice*. Oxford: Butterworth Heinemann.

Rolfe, G., Freshwater, D. and Jasper, M. (2001) *Critical Reflection for Nurses and the Caring Professions: A user's guide*. Basingstoke: Palgrave – now Palgrave Macmillan.

Rose, K. (2000) Counselling as a product or a process? *Psychodynamic Counselling*, **3**(4): 387–400.

Roth, A. and Fonaghy, P. (1996) *What works for whom? A critical review psychotherapy research*. London: The Guildford Press.

Rowan, J. (1998) *Transformational Research*. In Clarkson, P. (ed.) *Counselling Psychology*. London: Routledge.

Stevens, P.M.J., Schade, A.L., Chalk, B. and Slevin, O.D.'A. (1993) *Understanding Research*. Edinburgh: Campion Press.

Conducting research in a clinical environment: Research questions, methods and support

Dawn Freshwater and Veronica Bishop

what kind of question is being asked ... does the evidence support the analysis; does it make sense? (Carr-Hill, 1997:186)

In the chapter we discuss the processes that are needed to create the design map of any research project, whatever its size or complexity. Advantages and disadvantages of various research paradigms are discussed and the research journey is described, from articulating the research question to deciding on the appropriate method(s), gaining ethics approval and securing good support mechanisms. Potential hazards are highlighted and strategies to overcome these offered.

Introduction

Fox (1982) saw little chance of nursing or any of the social disciplines ever being short of research problems to be investigated, but to the new researcher it could seem as if everything of particular interest has been done. Once you begin to think around the area which interests you, interest is essential if you are to see the work through to completion, ideas will flow and the opportunity exists for you to follow through with ideas or hunches that you have been gathering. Whether the aim is to investigate the care being given by literature search or to carry out a small project, to launch into a research degree or to plan a major study which will involve an entire multidisciplinary team with other health disciplines, statisticians and the like, there has to be clarity on what it is that is being investigated. This may sound very obvious, but simplicity at this stage – in the subject matter – is critical, and many fail at this early juncture. There are, as Stein (1999:112) found when he was planning his research study for a higher degree,

> a number of issues surrounding the process of refining research questions. For example, although the work ... may be very lengthy and complex it seemed clear that a simple idea had to be at its heart. Put another way, if the key issue cannot be summed up in a few sentences than there is probably a need to focus even more narrowly on some aspect.

Stein goes on to highlight that while it is not difficult to think of things one would *like* to know, it is not always so easy to see how such a question may be answered with any degree of conviction. Research questions can be derived from many sources, including practice, nursing theory, previous research studies, social concerns, ethical concerns and human concerns.

Identification of a research question

In the 1990s one of the authors was privileged to facilitate a World Health Organisation (WHO) primary care research workshop in Delhi. The goals of the workshop were that participants should identify and develop research questions related to the delivery of nursing and midwifery services and the most efficient and effective use of personnel resources towards the attainment of better health. For those attending the workshop the challenge lay not only in selecting a problem that was researchable and practicable, and within the local resources, but also in identifying the most appropriate methodology. Despite the academic qualifications of the workshop participants a great deal of discussion was required to pare down that which they would like to know into what was a feasible research question. Described by Bishop (1994) as the 'what' of nursing, or by Stevens et al. (1993) as the act of converting the research problem into a research subject, this is a process that occurs over time and is guided by the motivation and interests of the investigator as well as other external influences such as the requirements of funding bodies and employing organisations. The phrasing and the form of the research question will differ according to the preferred model of generating knowledge, that is, the scientist–practitioner model or the practitioner–researcher model. A question that draws upon the scientist–practitioner model, for example, might consist of variables and the relationship that exists between them, implying the possibilities for empirical testing, while a question based in the practitioner–researcher model might be phrased as an open-ended aim or a description of the focus on enquiry.

Ovretveit (1990) states that many problems in measurement are not caused by trying to measure things that cannot be measured but by trying to measure something that has not been properly specified. Specifying nursing activities in isolation is a challenge. Robinson (1992:64) puts this succinctly, stating that:

> It is anticipated that the next stage of nursing research will entail the scrutiny of methodologies appropriate to the study of complex, multi-factorial conditions which demand investigation in such evaluative research. It is predicated nevertheless that the controlling of a whole range of variables, which is a necessary feature of such methodologies, will not be sufficient to understand the rich complexity of nursing activities.

This rich complexity of nursing activities is what is so difficult to unpick when trying to focus on a specific aspect of care. For

---

Box 5.1 Possible questions

- How good is the pre-operative information when it is given fully and in a standardised way?
- What would you compare its effectiveness with?
- Can the staff who give the information be evaluated in their effectiveness?
- Can future information giving be planned and taught based on the findings?
- How do personality types, background and external support mechanisms affect patients' responses to the procedure?
- How does information given pre-operatively affect the physical outcomes in terms of analgesia, well-being and discharge.

example, imagine that you work on a female surgical unit and that you have noticed that some women seem to take the loss of a breast with some stoicism while others are far more distressed. You may wonder why there are such variations in response to a similar procedure. In thinking around this you may notice that the pre-operative information giving is patchy where you work and wonder if it could be improved. How effective is it at its best? Does it make much difference at all – is it time wasted when it is carried out? Are patients more upset if they have a partner, or less? Does their response depend on their social background, their past experiences, and so on? So what is your research question? From the quite small list just given there are several research questions and related issues, some of which can be seen in Boxes 5.1

Box 5.2 Possible issues

- Do I need to limit the study to a certain age group?
- How many of the selected population (patients undergoing mastectomy) need to be studied for valid, generalisable results?
- How do I ensure that the pre-operative care was standardised for all patients to be studied?
- How do I try to account for other variables like personality, family support, severity of diagnosis, background and so on?
- How do I standardise the information givers?
- Shall I measure the effectiveness of the information givers who have been trained against those who have not?
- What will be my criteria for effectiveness?
- What method of investigation will achieve a robust answer with the least difficulty?
- How much time have I got to carry this out?
- What are the cost implications?
- Do I need to simplify the whole thing?
- What help and resources do I need?

and 5.2. These relate mainly to a scientist–practitioner model of investigation. Lack of clarity about what the research is trying to achieve will produce sloppy research and the possibility of the researcher drowning in a sea of data with no clear end result – and potentially an unethical approach.

Ethics, research governance and the research question

Ethics are described as a set of moral principles that govern a person's behaviour or the conducting of an activity. Ethics are a part of a social context and the nurse's role in ethical conduct, whether in daily activities or in research is central to the philosophy of caring. It is this caring aspect that in any discipline must not be forgotten in the excitement of research processes, a fact that the eminent scientist Payne (1978) raised with his medical colleagues when he reminded them that they were primarily concerned with caring for people, and that the art of medicine should not be forgotten in the enthusiasm for scientific precision. The researcher has an ethical responsibility throughout the process of research to ensure that the work is carried out in accordance with the approved ethical proposal, that data are handled sensitively and, where necessary, in strict confidence. Once an ethics committee has approved a proposal the lead researcher has an obligation to ensure that the protocols are adhered to and that any proposed changes which may arise once the research journey is begun, as if often the case, are formally approved. This degree of accountability and associated responsibility is not to be taken lightly and applies just as much to the small project as to the grand scale research programme. In addition it is an area of growing concern for studies being undertaken with staff and carers as well as patients.

The move to involve the public in research processes, rather than use them merely as subjects from whom to collect data, is a difficult one. As Beresford (2003:45) states:

> User involvement in research and evaluation is ultimately an ideological and ethical not a technical issue. User involvement in research raises fundamental issues. It has far reaching implications; for what we may

> understand by research ethics, research governance and indeed research itself. User involvement in research is not a comfortable or cosy idea, as is sometimes still suggested.

He goes on to suggest that user or public involvement ' should not be regarded as an add-on to existing research approaches and strategies. Its potential to transform understandings of and approaches to research, means that we must seek to approach it critically, systematically and without prejudice.'

The government-led initiative of research governance is now becoming well documented (Focus, 2003) and has direct impact on NHS staff and academics. Clifford (2003:14) identifies that

> The NHS research governance standards have major implications for staff and student nurses working in university settings. It places an onus upon these groups to adhere to the research governance agenda at the point of care giving when working in clinical areas in the NHS ... Moreover, it raises specific challenges to the increasing number of nurses employed by universities but undertaking clinical research as they must adhere to NHS requirements.

She goes on to point out that a great deal of development work will need to be undertaken as, 'depending upon the organisation, research management in universities may differ in their require-ments and so place the researcher in the position of meeting the demands of two organisations'. Clifford contends that analysis of the Department of Health research governance agenda along-side university standards for good practice in research does not reveal major difference in philosophy, but 'rather the emphasis on organisational models for managing and monitoring research may differ'. Clearly it is important that academic staff are famil-iar with local directives, not only for their own research activities but also in their supervision of students carrying out research in clinical areas in the NHS.

Literature search

It is at this stage that the investigator might interact with the literature as indicated in Chapter 4. Literature can be accessed through libraries (a kindly librarian is worth their weight in gold) and through web sites. Use key words to access the subject, and as you read through papers cross-reference the references, keeping an index. This will be invaluable to you as you progress in your work – a small effort which pays great dividends. Evaluate what other people have studied in a similar field, check the methods used and populations studied as this can expand what is available to you. Once a slightly firmer picture of the topic and appropriate methods has been delineated it is worth testing it against your clinical and academic peers. This is a sure way to be brought back to earth is you have been flying in esoteric circles. Taking your more refined thinking to colleagues who have some experience in research to obtain their views may also help to develop the focus, particularly in relation to appropriate methodology for the questions. We cannot overemphasise that time spent in the early stages of refining the question and considering methodological options will be more than repaid in the later stages of the work.

Selection of appropriate methodology

Those things that are the most measurable are not always of the greatest value, as Seedhouse (1988) observed. It is certainly much easier to measure those things that can be measured without difficulty; however, to quote Marinker (1994:12) 'it must be remembered that when facts are determined by the stakeholders the research bias may be as much in the questions posed as in the answers obtained'.

Health care professionals carry within them an enormous bank of knowledge, in part learned formally, in part gleaned through life experiences, and in part developed almost without consciousness as the formal learning and the learner move together in a particular environment, honing skills, sharpening awareness, becoming an expert professional. Ask a nurse if he or she has ever arrived at a ward to visit a friend or relative and made an instant positive or negative decision about the quality of care being provided and he or she will usually nod in agreement. What is being measured, assuming that on the face of it there are no glaring failings to be seen? And are we correct? Usually the answer is yes. Polanyi (1967) captures this implicit knowing saying that people often know more than they can tell – their knowledge cannot be put into words but is tacit knowledge. However, in order to have a better understanding of what we do, to learn how to improve and to meet the challenges of a dynamic society, it is important to try to articulate the art of caring into some form of language that is both representative and credible.

The established scientific community sees itself as the very paradigm of institutionalised rationality but is moving slowly away from its consideration that the process of elimination (the null hypothesis) is not necessarily the only way to generate knowledge. Bishop (2001), while considering that it may be too dangerous and expansive to promote totally, refers to the need for some degree of an academic habeas corpus – that is, that an idea may be considered sound until proven otherwise. There are numerous research texts and papers that outline the methodological approaches available. This chapter does not aim to rehearse this literature, rather we seek to raise awareness of the need to select an appropriate method when attempting to address a research question.

Below we briefly outline some of the main methods, building upon the models and issues presented in Chapter 4. While the methods presented here are by no means exhaustive and do not discount other paradigms they have been tried and tested in the investigation of nursing and social issues and as such could prove useful to the researcher in reaching an understanding of the strengths and weaknesses of the various routes to enquiry. At this point it is worth recalling the words of Popper, a prominent British philosopher who in 1968 made reference to the 'ultimate sources' of human knowledge writing: 'I propose to assume, instead, that no such ideal sources exist – no more than ideal rulers – and that all sources are liable to lead us into error at times' (p. 25).

Quantitative research

Quantitative research has its origins in positivism – put simply this means that there is a built-in assumption that there is an objective reality that can be measured or observed in some way. The types of data derived from quantitative research are usually numeric and linked to the natural and physical sciences. Quantitative research designs have high scientific credibility and are generally used in conditions that lend themselves to very specific issues where variables can be controlled or accounted for. Where quantifiable data are available they should, as a general rule, be taken into account as they may substantiate and verify findings obtained from other instruments used in the study. For further information it is recommended that the reader obtains a copy of the peer-reviewed paper by Seers and Crichton (2001).

Qualitative research

Qualitative research is based in the interpretivist paradigm in which knowledge is produced inductively. In other words qualitative research can be defined as research that produces findings not arrived at by means of quantification. Many qualitative researchers share a humanistic philosophy, however their individual beliefs originate from within the discipline in which they operate and are reflected in the way they research. Nursing and the social sciences, in order to improve their effectiveness, need to understand person-centred issues such as personal perceptions, experiences and individual knowledge. This is highlighted by Bailey (2001:551), who states that 'Without knowledge of what illness and healthcare mean to people of and of how lives are changed, we are left groping or insensitive about what it means to care for people'.

Many narrative researchers concur on this point, most notably Frank (2000) who espouses the value of narrative in understanding the meaning of illness and health. However, as Bailey (2001) and Freshwater and Rolfe (2001) stress, this approach to enquiry must, none the less, involve the essentials of rigorous investigation, including systematic procedures, theorising and a critical stance. This is not without its difficulties, but the advantages of a carefully planned qualitative study are many (Holloway and Fulbrook, 2001). Standard techniques used in carrying out qualitative research are life history research, interviewing, the use of analogue scales – usually on a 0–10 basis, validated questionnaires and a variety of therapeutic approaches originating in the humanities (Picard, 2002; Parker, 2002; Wagner, 2002). A recent major innovation in taking nursing and social science enquiry further is through critical reflexivity (Freshwater and Rolfe, 2001;

Alvesson and Skoldberg, 2000). Based on the concept of critical reflection on practice, critical reflexivity is less a technique and more an ability. Demanding that practice be called into question, it is the ability to combine immersion with critical distance.

Action research

LeMay and Lathlean (2001) argue that action research, a relatively attractive paradigm for nursing and health care in research terms, has the potential 'to contribute to the development of knowledge as well as to facilitate and evaluate change' (p. 509) and as such it deserves a mention here. This method of investigation may be seen as being at the other end of the scientific spectrum from quantitative study and is only now gaining academic respectability. A definition offered by Carr and Kemmis (1986:162) is that 'Action research is simply a form of self-reflective enquiry undertaken by participants in social situations in order to improve the rationality and justice of their own practices, their understanding of those practices, and the situations in which the practices are carried out'. Certainly the use of this method of research can be seen as reaching a state of maturity, evidenced by the *British Medical Journal* commissioning a paper on the subject (Meyer, 2000) and by the National Co-ordinating Centre for Service Delivery and Organisation actively supporting its use in application for research funding (Meyer, 2001). Many practice development projects are now based on action research and are used in conjunction with critical reflexivity, known as reflexive action research (Freshwater, 2000; Freshwater and Rolfe, 2001; Rolfe, Freshwater and Jasper, 2001; Alvesson and Skoldberg, 2000).

Triangulation

When more than one method of investigation is used it is called triangulation. Triangulation can take place both within methods and across methods. An example of this is where a study has used a quantifiable measure, such as weight of a patient, plus a questionnaire on their eating habits (which is not necessarily verifiable) and analysis of qualitative interviews. There are those who do not advocate triangulation, claiming that different approaches are based on differing ideologies and philosophies (Leininger, 1992), however Seale (1999) maintains that ideological principles can be maintained even across different perspectives.

Designing the research

Within the rough categories outlined above there are many research designs with specific characteristics. The research design is the map of the territory, that is to say it is a plan that governs the conduct of the research, albeit being dynamic and flexible. Factors affecting the design of the research revolve mainly around the research question and the investigators knowledge of the research topic and methodologies. Research designs that fall into the scientist practitioner model include:

- descriptive
- experimental
- quasi-experimental
- correlational

Practitioner researcher designs vary but may include:

- phenomenology
- grounded theory
- case study
- hermeneutics
- ethnomethodology
- critical or emancipatory research
- action research
- philosophical analysis.

The research design has significant implications for the manner in which the data are collected and analysed. Data can be collected in various ways, using different research instruments even within the same research question. Other factors to be taken into consideration when designing the blueprint for the research include the size of the sample population or the number of artefacts to be examined, the time available and ethical issues. Data collection moves through several different phases, however the key to the explanation and dissemination of the findings are the circumstances in which the data were collected and the processes that surrounded them. To this end we would recommend, as many other writers do, keeping a research diary. Indeed for some methods, such as critical and emancipatory research, it is a vital part of the data. Essentially the method of data collection takes place either in the form of observation, measurement or questioning, each demanding its own mode of analysis whether this be factual or process driven. Carr-Hill (1997:186) makes an important point when he succinctly states:

> The dichotomy between quantitative and qualitative research is overplayed. There are several important issues: what kind of question is being asked; how has the research been designed and who designs it (whichever package of methods is used); does the evidence support the analysis; does it make sense?

Dissemination

Keeping a research diary has more than one benefit. If the research process has been recorded in a journal then the pulling together of a research report or a paper for publication should not be too difficult. Whilst much will have changed over the time that the research has taken place journal entries serve as reminders for deviations from the original blueprint, how one handled sensitive situations and generally the highs and lows of the process. The importance of making the findings of research study open to public scrutiny cannot be over emphasised and this is addressed more fully in Chapter 10.

Appropriate support and supervision

Whatever career you choose it is important to embrace the concept of lifelong learning, and rather than see this as a burden to be carried until you win the lottery see it as your right. There is no mystery to learning and no monopoly of its ownership. It is now the right (and indeed responsibility) of every nurse to learn both in the daily clinical routine and within a properly supervised academic environment. There are of course differing learning styles and it is important to decide what method best suits you as an individual learner, and when looking for a supervisor try to find a suitable match. Additional to the conventional educational systems there is now, as a result of *Working Together – Learning Together* (DoH, 2001), the option to pursue professional development through electronic learning. This document outlines the role which e-learning should play within the NHS, stating that by December 2002 all NHS employer organisations should have had in place a local five-year e-learning strategy and capability in line with national Information for Health and NHS Information Authority plans and targets. To this end a Nursing Leadership Project rolled out the largest national e-learning project for clinical staff in 2001 in order to ascertain the readiness of both clinical staff and organisations within the NHS for e-learning (Dawes, 2002).

Whether you are a novice researcher, a novice in your post or an accepted expert in your field you need to keep abreast of changes to be able to assimilate and critique them and their relevance to clinical practice. One method of doing this is through critical reflection on practice, facilitated within the environment of either clinical supervision, research supervision, mentorship or journal clubs. This is lifelong learning and can best be done in good company! Find a peer group, or form one, network within your speciality – take the opportunity presented by attending conferences, use email and the web to dialogue with international colleagues. Having found or developed a network for peer review you then need to pick a supervisor (either clinical, research or both) who can challenge you without knocking into hierarchical barriers or creating an uncomfortable power dynamic. Clinical supervision is integral to the document *Making a Difference* (DoH, 1999) and will, we hope, gradually become a part of the nursing culture, changing it from one of didacticism to one of shared learning with a practice-based research philosophy (Bishop, 1998:2001). It is about providing a facilitative, instructive and constructive approach to an educated workforce, and to that end, as Driscoll (2000:196) notes, clinical supervision will support the clinical governance view that there is no end point in learning. A large accumulation of writings on clinical supervision highlights its importance in turning nurses around from 'doers' into 'thinking doers' (Rolfe et al., 2001). Those wishing to pursue this subject further will find suggested reading at the end of this book.

When choosing a research supervisor accessibility is a key concern, as is their background. The supervisor should be scientifically qualified to an appropriate level in order to challenge and guide the neophyte researcher and ideally should have an interest and rapport with their supervisee. Rafferty (1999:v) notes that 'serving a research apprenticeship is a daunting, dizzying, as well as a developmental experience. At times it seems more akin to the tale of the sorcerer's apprentice; overwhelming and out of control!' Clearly the role of the supervisor is pivotal to keeping the research journey within as safe a territory as possible, and cannot be underestimated, a view endorsed by others (Bishop, 1999; Philips and Pugh, 1987). However, the supervisory relationship is also influential in the maintenance of interest, excitement and challenge, a difficult balance to achieve. Sometimes this very vital relationship is taken for granted, and the inherent expectations are not voiced – indeed may not be shared. This is not a time for assumptions. It is important to make your expectations clear at the outset to avoid setting the supervisor up to fail. At times it will be the supervisor's subject knowledge or technical expertise that fulfils a need, at other times it is about being supportive, rewarding, challenging or simply bolstering sagging motivation and self-doubt (Millar 1999:79). Miller, as an academic supervisor, compares the experience as not so much a casual Sunday car outing but more like a car rally, with its peaks and troughs of emotion, the researcher at the wheel and the supervisor working as part of the team.

A contract, informal or formal, should be set up between both supervisor and supervisee and adhered to. This, while accommodating different styles of work and personality, will produce a greater likelihood of a happy outcome. It is quite acceptable to have more than one supervisor, each knowing of the other, and indeed in multidisciplinary work would be essential to bring the breadth of expertise required to the study. Many academic institutions insist on a supervisory team for students registered on research degrees, believing this to be of mutual benefit. For any research degree supervisors must be approved by the host university or educational institution, which can bring with it problems if suitable candidates are in short supply. It can be helpful here to have already approached, informally, suitably qualified and willing academics at other institutions and to seek collaborative arrangements formally, if necessary.

Conclusion

In conclusion, as stated at the outset of this chapter, there is little chance of there being any shortage of problems to be investigated in the health services, and the opportunities to pursue areas of interest have never been better. However, in this chapter we have sought to identify potential hazards for the novice researcher, and to highlight strategies to avoid or overcome these.

Key points

- Clarity of purpose and method is essential to good research.
- Choose a subject which will maintain your interest.
- Peer groups may help to foster critical practice.
- Dissemination is integral to good research practices.

References

Alvesson, M. and Skoldberg, K. (2000) *Reflexive Methodology*. London: Sage.

Bailey, C. (2001) Revisiting qualitative inquiry: interviewing in nursing and midwifery research. *Nursing Times Research*, **6**(1).

Beresford, P. (2003) User involvement in research: exploring the challenge. *Nursing Times Research*, **8**(1): 36–46.

Bishop, V. (1994) Prevention and primary health care delivery challenges. In Fitzpatrick, J.J., Stevenson, J.S. and Polis, N.S. (eds) *Nursing Research and its Utilisation*. New York: Springer.

Bishop, V. (1998) Editorial. N*ursing Times Research*, **6**: 484.

Bishop, V. (1999) *Clinical supervision in Practice. Some questions, answers and guidelines*. Basingstoke: Macmillan – now Palgrave Macmillan.

Bishop, V. (2001) Professional development and clinical supervision. In Bishop, V. and Scott, I. (eds) *Challenges in clinical practice. Professional developments in nursing*. Basingstoke: Palgrave – now Palgrave Macmillan.

Carr, W. and Kemmis, S. (1986) *Becoming critical: education, knowledge and action research*. London: Falmer.

Carr-Hill, R. (1997) Commentary: Choosing between qualitative and quantitative approaches. *Nursing Times Research*, **2**(3): 186.

Clifford, C. (2003) Research Governance: The Challenge. *Nursing Times Research*. **8**(1): 7–16.

Dawes, D. (2002) A pilot study to assess the case for e-learning in the NHS. *NTResearch*, **7**(6): 428–43.

DoH (Department of Health) (1999) *Making a Difference. Strengthening the Nursing Midwifery and Health Visiting contribution to health and healthcare*. London: DoH.

DoH (Department of Health) (2001) *Working Together – Learning Together*. London: DoH.

Driscoll, J. (2000) *Practising clinical supervision. A reflective approach*. London: Ballière.

Focus (2003) Research Governance. *NTResearch*, **8**(1): 7–57.

Fox, D.J. (1982) *Fundamentals of Research in Nursing*. Crofts, East Norwalk: Appleton-Century.

Frank, A. (2000) The standpoint of story teller. *Qualitative Health Research*, **10**(28): 354–65.

Freshwater, D. (2000) *Transformatory Learning in Nurse Education*. Portsmouth: Nursing Praxis International.

Freshwater, D. and Rolfe, G. (2001) Critical Reflexivity: A politically and ethically engaged research method for nursing. *NTResearch*, **6**(1): 526–37.

Holloway, I. and Fulbrook, P. (2001) Revisiting qualitative inquiry. Interviewing in nursing and midwifery research. *NTResearch*, **6**(1): 539–50.

Leininger, M. (1992) Current issues, problems and trends to advance qualitative paradigmatic research methods for the future. *Qualitative Health Research*, **2**(4): 392–415.

Le May, A. and Lathlean, J. (2001) Action research: A design with potential. *NTResearch*, **6**(1): 502–9.

Marinker, M. (1994) *Controversies in Health Care Policies: Challenges to Practice*. London: BMJ Publishing Group.

Meyer, J. (2000) Using qualitative methods in health related research. *British Medical Journal*, **320**: 178–81.

Meyer, J. (2001) Service Delivery and Organsiation: The Case for Action Research. In Fulop, N., Allen, P., Black, N. and Clarke, A. (eds) *Methods for studying the delivery and organisation of health services*. London: Routledge.

Millar, R. (1999) Supervisor's comments. In Bishop, V. (ed.) *Working towards a research degree*. London: Emap and NTBooks.

Oxford University Press (1998) *New Oxford Dictionary*. Oxford: Oxford University Press.

Ovretveit, J. (1990) *Quality health services*. Middlesex: Brunel University.

Parker, M.E. (2002) Aesthetic Ways in day to day nursing. In Freshwater, D. (ed.) *Therapeutic Nursing*. London: Sage.

Payne, J.P. (1978) Ethical problems in clinical research and intensive care. Editorial, *British Journal of Anaesthesia*, **50**: 515–18.

Phillips, E.M. and Pugh, D. (1987) How to get a PhD: A handbook for students and their supervisors (3rd edn). Buckingham: Open University Press.

Picard, C. (2002) A praxis model of research for therapeutic nursing. In Freshwater, D. (ed.) *Therapeutic Nursing*. London: Sage.

Polanyi, M. (1967) *The Tacit Dimension*. Garden City, New York: Anchor.

Popper, K. (1968) *Conjectures and Refutations*. New York: Harper Torch Books.

Rafferty, A.M. (1999) Foreword. In Bishop, V. (ed.) *Working Towards a Research Degree*. London: Emap.

Robinson, J. (1992) NHS research and development towards the year 2000. Trent RHA 11th seminar.

Rolfe, G., Freshwater, D. and Jasper, M. (2001) *Critical Reflection for Nursing and the Caring Professions*. Basingstoke: Palgrave – now Palgrave Macmillan.

Seale, C. (1999) *The Quality of Qualitative Research*. London: Sage.

Seedhouse, D. (1988) *Ethics: The heart of health care*. London: Wiley.

Seer, K. and Crichton, N. (2001) Quantitative research: Designs relevant to nursing and healthcare. *Nursing Times Research*, **6**(1): 487–500.

Stein, B. (1999) Selecting a subject: problems and solutions. In Bishop, V. (ed.) *Working towards a research degree*. London: Emap.

Stevens, P.J.M., Scahde, A.L., Chalk, B. and Slevin, O.D.A. (1993) *Understanding Research*. Edinburgh: Campion.

Wagner, A.L. (2002) Nursing students' development of caring self through creative reflective practice. In Freshwater, D. (ed.) *Therapeutic Nursing*. London: Sage.

Part II

Professional Development for Careers in Research

Doctoral processes: The scholarly practitioner

Hugh McKenna and Kathleen Galvin

In this chapter the case is strongly made for doctoral study. In recent years the number of doctoral programmes for nursing has increased dramatically. In the United Kingdom alone there are almost eighty university schools of nursing and most have doctoral students. At its best a doctoral programme involves discovering and disseminating knowledge to benefit practice. In countries where nurses have been delayed in gaining admission to doctoral programmes the development of nursing knowledge has also been delayed. We describe the development of a diverse range of doctorates and discuss their relevance and contribution to the development of nursing and its practice.

Introduction

Members of any profession are best able to appreciate the essence of their discipline when their educational programme includes not only studying but also generating, challenging and testing the knowledge in their field (Lanara, 1994). Benz and Shapiro (1998:66) underline this idea in their conceptualisation of the role of 'scholarly practitioner'.

> Using professional practice and knowledge as a resource for the formulation and production of scholarly knowledge as well as for evaluating, testing, applying, extending, or modifying existing knowledge. It involves mastering procedures for generating knowledge, not only to create knowledge but as important, to become aware of the limits of knowledge.

Downs (1978, 1988) maintained that adequate preparation of doctoral students is among the most important and pressing educational issues facing nursing, for nursing must depend upon this group of individuals for the critical and creative study of its science. In this chapter we describe the historical development of doctoral education in nursing, highlight key features of today's

UK postgraduate sector, and describe the different doctorates available from UK universities and the process involved in admission and examination of a doctorate. To help the reader use terminology to label types of doctorates, since the nomenclature is not clear in the general literature, the PhD by thesis we term 'traditional doctorate' and the range of doctorates with taught and thesis components 'professional doctorates'.

Historical perspective

Doctoral education in nursing had its birth in the United States of America. According to Grace (1978) the historic progression towards doctorate studies for American nurses had three stages. In the early part of the twentieth century a small number of nurses studied for the Doctor of Education degree (EdD), the most famous of which was at Teachers' College in Columbia University, New York. Doctor of Philosophy degrees (PhD) became common and a substantial number of US universities introduced Doctor of Nursing Science degrees (DSc). In some cases the DSc was introduced because the university authorities did not allow a fledgling discipline like nursing to offer PhDs.

Lash (1987) pointed out that in the US there were five main types of doctorate programmes favoured by nurses. These are Doctor of Philosophy (PhD), Doctor of Nursing Studies (DNS); Doctor of Nursing Science (DSc); Doctor of Nursing and Doctor of Education (DE). Unlike the traditional European PhD, which was thesis based, all these US programmes had a substantial taught component and can be termed 'professional doctorates'.

In the early 1950s US nurse education moved almost entirely into universities. The new university undergraduate courses could not be sustained through being composed entirely of anatomy, physiology, biology, psychology and sociology. Nurse teachers had to begin to teach nursing, and this meant an increasing number had to research and philosophise on the substance and essence of nursing. Another reason was the desire to move away from the previously pervading medical model. In addition nurses were mostly women and as a result of the Second World War women were having a greater influence in society and were taking

Table 6.1 Development Trajectory of Doctorates in Nursing in the USA

Year	Number of doctoral programmes
1954	2
1977	17
1985	29
1990	50
1999	70, with 16 in development

on more high-profile roles. Therefore, from the 1950s onwards, there was rapid development in US nurse doctoral programmes (see Table 6.1) (Anderson, 2000).

While this seems a large number of programmes, in the 1980s there were 1.5 million American nurses, but only 0.16 per cent had studied at doctoral level (Anderson, 2000). The key influences for this rapid development were growth in academic courses and the need for doctoral-prepared academic staff to teach on undergraduate and graduate programmes (Lancaster, 1984).

The US doctorate programmes that emerged reflected the stages of discipline development and were influenced by the structure of the US academy and the American health care system. Therefore they changed in purpose and curriculum structure over time, reflecting the demand for a wide range of specific roles including undergraduate and postgraduate programmes and a mix of clinically focused and academically orientated curricula. This presents a very unclear differentiation between the aims and terminology of the range of doctorates with a research or practice focus or both (Lancaster, 1984; Ziemer, et al., 1992).

Furthermore in the US there is no clear distinction between professional doctorates and the PhD, although Newman distinguishes the 'academic' doctorate from the doctorate for professional practice preparation (Newman, 1975). On close examination of their curricula their aims and philosophy are not clearly distinguished and differences between the dissertations are not well defined (Lancaster, 1984). Both types require similar amounts of academic credit and present a similar modularised form covering research methods, theory development, clinical specialisation, teaching, leadership and research dissertation

(INDEN, 2002, Ketefian, Neves and Gutierrez, 2001). Further evidence of poor differentiation has been provided by Downs (1989) who reviewed 43 DNS and traditional PhD programmes. Her findings reflected Lancaster's (1984) conclusions but also indicated that DNS programmes tended to have more clinical hours whereas the PhD had more emphasis on research methods and analysis. Hudacek and Carpenter (1998) have also reported that students perceive that different programmes act as preparation for different roles. They explored the perceptions of 401 students from 54 US PhD, DNS and DEd programmes. PhD students perceived their degree as preparation for roles as researchers. This was statistically different from students undertaking professional doctorate degrees who perceived that their course was preparation for roles as practitioners, administrators and educators.

In contrast to the United States, the availability of doctoral education for nurses in the UK is a relatively recent phenomenon, occurring sixty years post North American developments. Here, doctoral education for nurses did not go through the first of Graces' three stages (1978). Rather it commenced with a small number of nurses undertaking traditional PhDs in related fields, such as education, sociology and psychology. In many cases these students investigated nurses rather than nursing and contributed more to the academic disciplines of sociology and psychology than to nursing *per se*. Furthermore, many non-nurse sociologists and psychologists gained their PhD by studying the nursing profession.

In the 1970s the number of UK universities offering nursing PhD degrees could be counted in single figures. Only in the 1990s did nurses begin to undertake doctoral study in significant numbers. After a comprehensive search of the literature, indexes of theses and research libraries, Traynor estimated that in 1997 there were three hundred nurses with PhD degrees in the UK (Traynor and Rafferty, 1998) However, as nurse education has moved into the university sector these numbers are increasing exponentially.

As distinct from the US system, UK PhD students do not follow a taught programme. Rather they adhere to a European model of study, culminating in a research thesis (traditional PhD). Commonly, the entry requirement is an undergraduate degree. While three years' full-time study is preferable and available, most tend to undertake their doctorate part-time over a five-year period. This is probably due to the lack of funding for full-time study.

Five years is a long time, and when balanced with personal responsibilities and full-time employment the drop-out rate from part-time PhDs in many disciplines is high (UKCGE, 2002). Furthermore, by the time the student completes and publishes his or her findings seven years may have passed and the impact on knowledge and practice may be reduced considerably. However, recently a range of new-style doctorate programmes has been developed in the UK which may potentially offer some solutions to these problems.

Types of doctoral degrees and the current UK postgraduate context

Currently in the UK there are a number of ways that nurses can study for a doctoral degree. These include the traditional PhD by thesis, the PhD by published work and the professional doctorate. The nature of each of these types of programme is discussed later.

The emergence of professional nursing doctorates in the UK took place in a context of rapid development of new-style doctorates in a range of disciplines. The major driver was to enhance the contribution that postdoctoral graduates could have to enterprise and business and to make doctorates more compatible with the needs of practice. Bourner, Bowden and Laing, (2001) reported that the development of these new approaches to doctoral curricula was slow, with the first being introduced as recently as 1992 (the EdD at Bristol and, in the same year, Engineering at Warwick, Wales, Manchester and UMIST). There was exponential development over the next six years and by 1998 there were 109 programmes available in 19 subjects. It is of note that Bourner et al., reported that five subjects accounted for most of the new professional doctorate programmes (education, psychology, medicine, business administration and engineering). It is no surprise that these are all practice-focused disciplines. Of note is that the first doctorate in Nursing Science in Europe was established at the University of Ulster in 1995 (Boore, 1996).

The contextual features for these developments include:

- an overall increase in part-time study in the UK (HESA, 1999)
- the desire by students to be engaged in practice or industry while studying at doctoral level
- personal development and project work being key motivational factors in doctorate study (Becher, 1994)
- professional doctor or nursing science programmes have modular structures reflecting requirements placed on universities (Bourner et al., 2001), contrasting sharply with traditional doctorates which lack structure and have been criticised as too narrow and not applied (Booth, 2001)
- the synergy between practice development, personal development and discipline development represent the new 'heart' of doctoral study in practice disciplines (Bourner et al., 2001; Galvin and Carr 2003).

PhD by thesis

In the UK the PhD by thesis is a research-based training and qualification. Its foundation is a sustained period engaged in research which makes an original contribution to knowledge (UK Council for Graduate Education, 2002). Therefore doctoral programmes that require a thesis do so as a means of preparing future researchers. Historically formal guidance and structure were lacking and the process was very much dependent upon the relationship between the student and supervisor. The supervisor reviews the proposed project for suitability as a PhD or a Masters of Philosophy project. Following this, the supervisor and student discuss the feasibility of the study, for example, availability of equipment and resources to support the proposed study, subject availability, and whether ethical permission will be possible. Commonly the proposal will be formally peer reviewed by a university research committee.

Because the traditional PhD is by thesis only it is not a requirement that students attend lectures or undertake examinations or coursework. Increasingly, however, PhD students are encouraged to attend lectures on research methods and theory. More UK universities are establishing research graduate schools where students are supported and have regular seminars on key skills such as:

- the use of quantitative and qualitative data analysis software
- presentation software
- writing for publication
- writing grant proposals
- presenting at conferences.

Quality provision of doctoral programmes is guided by seven codes of practice from the UK Quality Assurance Agency (QAA, 1999). These are:

I.   General principles and research environment
II. Promotional information and selection and admission
III. Enrolment, registration, induction and information
IV. Approval of project and skills training
V.   Supervision
VI. Examination,Feedback, appeals and complaints
VII. Evaluation

The culmination of a traditional PhD is a research thesis of approximately 80,000–100,000 words indicating sustained independent effort on the part of the student, that a process of research training has occurred, and that the student has made a substantial contribution to the subject area. Students are encouraged to submit on time and the Higher Education Funding Council strictly monitors UK university completion times and rates. Historically completion rates have been varied in some disciplines with some departments achieving only one-third of student completions, mainly because students never submitted a thesis for examination (UKCGE, 2002). Recently The British Academy (for Humanities and the Social Sciences) undertook a review of graduate studies in the humanities and the social sciences and identified many complex factors contributing to a crisis in numbers and quality of students. The review showed that overall numbers and completions are declining due to financial disincentives, unattractive academic career paths, rigidity of traditional PhD structure and barriers for mature professionals to undertake PhD study. These factors are highly pertinent to nurses and indicate the need for new enticements to encourage PhD registration and completion. Such enticements could include increased availability of postgraduate funding awards, more flexible PhD study, collaborative ventures between universities, support for complex projects (for instance it is difficult in nursing to undertake a complex intervention study single handed for the purposes of a PhD), and greater opportunity for part time students.

Mason and McKenna (1995) explored the problems and difficulties involved in undertaking a nursing PhD. Many students found the 'non-taught' nature of this degree a lonely and frustrating endeavour and non-completion was a major problem. Although full-time students lacked financial resources for programme completion they can earn extra money by undertaking demonstrations and tutorials within the university. However, a sponsoring or grant-awarding body may place restrictions on what a student can be asked to do outside the boundaries of their project.

PhD by published work

A PhD by published work requires the student to have a portfolio of scholarly work consisting of a number of papers published in international, peer-reviewed journals on a specific topic. Individuals may choose this route because they are unable, for a variety of reasons, to undertake a PhD in the traditional manner. For instance, a senior nurse academic may have a busy head of department role and, while they never registered for a PhD, they may have, over a number of years, published research and theoretical papers with a particular focus. As alluded to above, a PhD represents sustained independent effort, research training and a significant contribution to the field. It is possible that this senior staff member has met these criteria, especially if expert peer reviewers have judged the publications to be of the right standard to be published in peer reviewed journals.

Normally the PhD by published work portfolio is composed of an introductory theoretical chapter followed by a number of published peer-reviewed papers, each relating to the research topic. A final chapter concludes the portfolio and documents how the author has expanded the knowledge base of the field. As with the PhD by thesis, an oral examination takes place and, if successful, the individual is awarded a PhD. While this variation of the PhD is becoming increasingly available some universities restrict eligibility to individuals who are staff or have some visiting capacity to the university.

This approach to doctoral study is similar to that in Sweden, where a doctorate is composed of a thesis consisting of a number of (five to six) peer-reviewed papers 'topped and tailed' by introductory and concluding chapters. There are particular challenges in supporting the development of PhDs by publication. These include the credibility of the original contribution to new knowledge, which in nursing may draw upon critical reflective analysis of complex problems in practice and non-traditional data. The examination of new forms of theses present challenges in the preparation of supervisors and examiners and in achieving some consensus about broadly stated assessment criteria. Quality criteria for doctoral study are difficult to articulate (INDEN, 2002) and the existing 'gold standard' is not homogeneous between disciplines or between the range of doctoral programmes (UKCGE, 1996, 1998).

Professional doctorates in nursing

Currently much discussion is occurring in the UK about the introduction of professionally taught doctoral programmes for nurses. These doctoral programmes are similar to the US Doctor in Nursing Science (professional doctorate) degree programmes and are stimulating interest in Europe for the following reasons.

To most academics in Europe doctoral education means PhD study. However, the traditional PhD has not always strengthened the links between research, theory and practice. Invariably PhD students know a great deal about the literature pertaining to their topic and they can discuss their method at length and in great depth. However, the application of their findings to practice or future research is often a matter for the briefest consideration. In contrast the professional doctorate focuses specifically on the theory, practice and research linkage.

University integration

Within the past ten years nurse education in the Europe has entered the university sector. Neophyte nurse academics realise that having a successful career in this new environment necessitates gaining a doctoral degree. However, they are employed to teach nursing and they accept that it is sensible to ensure that their doctoral thesis expands the boundaries of knowledge in that field. Consequently a cadre of nurses has begun to consider professional doctoral routes, where nursing knowledge, nursing scholarship and the essence of nursing are given equal weight with research methods and techniques.

The nurse consultant role

Within recent years there has been an increase in the number of nurse consultants in the UK. These are senior roles with a 50 per cent practice and service development facet and 50 per cent leadership, education and evaluation facet (Guest et al., 2001). The initiative was supported by Tony Blair, the British Prime Minister, and was a means whereby expert nurses were able to plan a career without having to leave the clinical area and enter nurse management or nurse education. Currently there are over 250 nurse consultants in the UK with high-level research, practice development and leadership expertise. They have the potential to contribute to the development of evidence-based practice.

With its emphasis on integrating practice, theory and research, the professional doctorate is seen as an appropriate qualification for the nurse consultant role. Galvin and Carr (2002) undertook a survey of 200 consultant nurses and midwives by written invitation via the Department of Health. There was a 22.55 per cent response rate ($n = 45$). Nine were currently undertaking a doctorate and 36 had a master's degree. Twenty-one thought that a doctorate was very important to underpin their role, four were undecided and, interestingly, seven thought that a doctorate would not support their current role. Of the nine undertaking a doctorate two were undertaking a traditional programme, three a professional doctorate of nursing science and three a doctorate of education. (There was one non-response to this item.) As might be expected eight were undertaking their doctorate on a part-time basis, two were self-funding and seven were funded by their employer. While the data it is limited it seems that a small proportion of consultant nurses are prepared to doctorate level and a proportion are undertaking doctorates; but is it feasible to study for a doctorate and undertake a consultant role? It may be that future practitioners who aspire to be consultant nurses will be the key group taking up these programmes.

As indicated above, the first professional doctorate programme in the UK began in 1994 at the University of Ulster. Its establishment was a laborious process that included different layers of stringent validation and review (Boore, 1996). Applicants were carefully screened to ensure that their motivation for applying to the programme was to contribute to nursing rather than simply to gain an academic ticket for career purposes. Since 1994 a number of other UK universities have introduced professional doctorates in nursing (for example, Swansea, Northumbria, Sheffield, Nottingham and Southampton).

The admission, process and submission stages for these programmes are similar to that of the traditional PhD. All have a thesis ranging from 40,000 to 80,000 words. The main difference is that professional doctorate students attend classes and submit coursework. The students tend to be clinicians who want to remain in practice and have ambitions to become nurse consultants or hold joint appointment between a clinical area and a university department. They are attracted to the camaraderie and debate that being in a class group engenders and they need the discipline of coursework milestones rather than the academic loneliness of what they perceive to be the traditional PhD route, an observation borne out in feedback from students (Galvin and Carr, 2002). In addition, by its nature, scientific knowledge quickly becomes outdated and doctoral education has to be about process and outcome as well as substantive content. The following assumptions by West (1966) illustrate this perfectly:

- Only a small portion of the current body of knowledge can be taught in the prescribed period of time.
- Much of the knowledge that will be employed in the students' future career is not known today and therefore cannot be taught.

- Not all that is taught is learned.
- A portion of what is learned will soon be obsolete.
- Of that which is learned, much is quickly forgotten.
- A small part of what is taught is error (not research based).

In addition, the current context suggests that personal development in preparation for postdoctoral leadership means that doctorates have transformative aims and that personal growth and expertise development as well as research training are important features of doctoral study.

Most UK universities that have adopted the professional nursing doctorate approach have accepted that the educational challenge is to endow students with a clear sense of purpose and a lifetime love for expanding their intellectual horizons with regard to the substance of nursing. Students are encouraged to recognise themselves as emergent scientists and appreciate the significance of the development of scholarly endeavours.

Attempts are made to enrich the student with the ability to think critically, to identify the gaps in nursing knowledge, to search for truth without prejudice, to take risks with ideas, and to be creative and imaginative in solving problems. In addition, the students acquire the ability and desire to present their work to their contemporaries and to accept critical comments without intense feelings of personal attack.

Students gain epistemological and ontological insights and are involved in seminar work that takes them along the continuum from identifying interesting phenomena in practice to formulating and testing concepts and theoretical propositions. They explore knowledge of other disciplines to identify new paradigms and methodologies that may generate new nursing knowledge.

As recommended by Meleis (1981), knowledge within doctoral programmes is explored epistemologically in relation to its origins, analytically in relation to its theoretical components and critically in terms of its significance and influence on the discipline of nursing.

The professional nursing doctorate seeks to take the doctoral student beyond what Benner (1984) referred to as expert practice to advanced practice. In Benner's study expert nurse participants could not always articulate why they knew certain things or why they practised in a particular way. The professional doctorate attempts to exploit tacit and explicit knowledge (Polanyi, 1958) so that successful graduates can articulate the reasons for their actions.

According to Benoliel (1977) scholars need to be able to move back and forth between the world of nursing practice and the abstract world of knowledge development. UK professional doctorates are founded on patient care being the seedbed for knowledge. Knowledge is generated from practice and has to be refined and returned to inform or be tested in practice. Therefore all applicants to these programmes must have easy access to patient care settings. This requirement is not merely to increase clinical expertise but to foster the linkage between theory, research and practice which is necessary for developing and testing nursing science.

The professional doctorate can be a challenge to academic staff and it is one that should be taken seriously. There must be a persistent vigilance to ensure that it does not become another series of taught modules where students master the content so that they can regurgitate it back in end of term assignments. According to Grace (1978) such a process is anathema to the independent and creative enterprise that needs to exist if a doctoral programme is to be of value in extending the boundaries of nursing knowledge. This is clearly a tension with the curriculum structure of modules, with inherent assessment, often a requirement of UK universities, driven by quality assurance mechanisms.

PhD versus professional doctorate

According to Lash (1987) and Grace (1978), North American nurses have difficulty differentiating between the PhD and the professional doctorates. Lash argued that these programmes are similar in that each has a theory strand, a research component and an integrative science component. He stated that the many similarities between these higher degrees made it difficult to tell them apart. In the UK the problems of differentiation between the PhD and the professional doctorate are not so acute. The former is an academic or research degree whereas a Doctorate of Nursing Science is a clinical and application of research degree. Several published papers support such a differentiation and indicate a need for multiple routes (Blancett, 1989; Seitz, 1987; McKenna and Cutcliffe, 2001) with varied purpose. The literature provides some differentiation between doctorate programmes but also indicates future challenges. These include differentiating their philosophy and the form and purpose of any thesis from that of the traditional PhD, being clear about intended impacts on students learning and its purpose for practice, and clarifying the aims of the doctorate's structure.

The mix of approaches to doctoral education is appropriate for the current stage of nursing development. Both degrees are rigorous, both are organised systematically in terms of length of programme and supervision. Both are concerned with the training of students in research methods, the generation of new knowledge and the presentation of primary research in the form of a dissertation. However the professional doctorate has the added benefits of structured support, peer group support and opportunities for personal development that are wider than a research training alone.

Therefore the major differences are in the delivery and the mission of the two programmes. The professional doctorate is a taught degree in which students have examination and coursework milestones. Professional doctorate students are encouraged to explore the substantive content of nursing knowledge and to become adept in a wide range of qualitative and quantitative methods. In contrast, PhD students may only study the method they are using for their study, and the final thesis may not pertain to practice or patient care. Doncaster and Thorne (2000) provided helpful terminology to describe two complementary roles underpinned by doctorates with different emphases: the 'professional scholar' and the 'scholarly professional'. The academic doctorate (PhD) aims to develop 'professional scholars' who will lead and support academic developments, research, push discipline edges and develop curricula, while the professional doctorate aims to produce 'scholarly professionals' who practice nursing with a sophisticated knowledge to inform practice that includes evidence, evaluation, critical reflection, practice development and research. Recently there has been evidence (Becher, Henkel and Kogan, 1994) in a range of disciplines away of a shift in the focus of doctoral study from considering research training as the main purpose of a PhD to project-focused work aimed at developing practice and personal development. This does not suggest that research training and practice focus are dichotomous but that in practice disciplines such as nursing a synergy must exist between the two.

Galvin and Carr (2002) reported perceptions of existing doctoral students that lend support to this differentiation. A purposive sample of 100 professional doctorate and 100 traditional doctorate students from four university departments was sampled. The response rate was 15.5 per cent ($n = 31$). In addition, a sample of nine consultant nurses who were undertaking doctorates were included in the analysis. Students ($n = 40$) were asked about their perceptions of the aims of their doctorate. These are summarised in Table 6.2.

Most ($n = 8$) perceived the key aims to be the generation of new knowledge or improving or contributing to the development of nursing practice; three perceived that preparation for research or personal needs were the key aim. Most (98 per cent) also agreed that the aim of doctoral study in nursing was 'new knowledge for improvement'. The majority were undertaking their PhD part time (Table 6.3).

The respondents identified what they perceived to be the most important attributes of doctorate courses. These were highly supportive systems and preparation for clinically focused research. Interestingly 41 per cent of respondents perceived exposure to multiple research methods and 62 per cent contact with other disciplines to be the least important feature (Table 6.4).

Table 6.2 Student perception of aim of doctorate

(Open response question)	Traditional PhD ($n = 10$)	Professional doctorate ($n = 18$)
Generation of new knowledge	2	6
Improving, contributing, developing nursing practice	6	6
Preparation for research	2	1
Developing theory	1	0
Personal aims	1	1
Raise profile of practice area	0	1

Table 6.3 Full- and part-time study

	Full-time study n = 16 (15%)	Part-time study n = 33 (82.5%)
Academic role	(1)	(11)
Consultant nurse	(1)	(8)
Clinical specialist	(1)	(7)
Research role	(3)	(3)
Other roles		(4)
missing n = 1		

The most important difficulties perceived by students were lack of opportunities to use skills in practice, lack of postdoctoral career structure, high volume of work and others' negative views of professional doctorates in nursing (Table 6.5).

The credibility of the doctorate title was seen as least important by 71 per cent of the sample. This is an interesting finding since it is an issue that course development teams often spend much time considering. The sample's aspirations following doctoral study are summarised in Table 6.6. There is a strong emphasis on practice-focused careers, with only 15 per cent aspiring to a career in an academic setting.

Table 6.4 Value of course characteristics as rated by respondents

	Most important (%)		Quite important (%)		Least important (%)	
Highly supportive systems	61.7	(21)	17.6	(6)	20.5	(7)
Exposure to multiple research methods	23.5	(8)	35.2	(12)	41.1	(14)
Preparation for clinically focused research	50.1	(17)	29.4	(10)	20.5	(7)
Contact with other disciples	14.7	(5)	23.5	(8)	61.7	(21)
Peer Support	32.3	(11)	41.1	(14)	26.4	(9)
Embedded in a research-active department	17.6	(6)	52.9	(18)	29.4	(10)

n = 34; missing = 6

Table 6.5 Rating of difficulties of doctoral programmes

	Most important (%)		Quite important (%)		Least important (%)	
Lack of opportunity to use skills in practice	7.14	(2)	71.4	(2)	21.4	(6)
Lack of post-doctoral career structure	14.2	(4)	67.8	(19)	17.8	(5)
High volume of work	67.8	(19)	21.4	(6)	10.7	(3)
Credibility of title	10.7	(3)	17.8	(5)	71.4	(20)
Negative views (by others) of professional doctorates	78.5	(22)	21.4	(6)	0	

$n = 28$, missing $= 12$

Table 6.6 Aspirations following completion of doctorate

Career development progression	(2)	5%
Consultant role	(3)	7.5%
Career in the academy	(6)	15%
Career in practice research	(8)	20%
Use of skills and knowledge in practice	(16)	40%

$n = 40$; missing (5) 12.5%

These findings, while from a small study, indicated that the motivation for doctoral study is clearly to contribute to practice and make an impact on patient care. However, the findings also showed that the need for expertise in a wide range of research methods and a broad skill set within a context of multiprofessional care delivery is not fully acknowledged by existing doctoral students. The findings also highlight the importance of structure and peer support in undertaking doctoral study in nursing.

Doctorate study process

Admission and supervision

There has been a change in the profile of students applying for admission to doctoral programmes (HESA, 1999) and processes within academic settings are varied, reflecting new types of students and programmes. The average age of UK students entering nursing doctoral programmes is 35. This is in contrast to those UK students who undertake doctoral study in the basic sciences such as biochemistry, where the average age on entry is 21 (Mason and McKenna, 1995). In the former, a doctoral degree is normally undertaken part time after a number of years in practice, education or both. In the latter the student commences a doctoral degree full time immediately following their primary degree. Recently younger nurses have been enrolling in UK doctoral programmes. This is due to a number of reasons, including the:

- availability of a small number of full-time research fellowships
- evolving career structures in universities
- advent of professional doctorates
- introduction of the clinical nurse consultant role, where a doctoral degree is perceived to be beneficial.

Ten to twenty years ago it was common for those UK nurses who wished to study at doctoral level to have identified a specific research topic before admission into the programme. After all, these nurses had spent many years in nursing practice or education and they knew precisely what they wanted to research. Furthermore they realised that they were going to work on the project for a number of years, consequently they selected a topic that held their interest.

Because the new university-based schools of nursing wanted to attract doctoral students, research supervisors often agreed to supervise on a range of topics. This was not a new phenomenon as it was always common for nurse tutors to teach a variety of topics across the curricula, often without the necessary expertise. More recently a new maturity is emerging where nurse academics are becoming more selective with regard to the research topics they will supervise. An emerging trend is for the supervisor to provide the topic and the research proposal and for the student to apply through a competitive process to undertake the work.

Another trend is mutual decision-making in supervisor and student selection. The student may check potential supervisors' credibility in the field, their publications, research grants and the number of doctoral students they have supervised to successful completion. Potential students may also speak with other students who have been supervised by the academic staff member. Therefore admission may be through a competitive or speculative process.

On entry to a doctoral programme a student is assigned to a research supervisor who meets certain criteria. Supervisors must:

- have a doctorate
- be expert in the topic
- have supervised other doctoral students to timely and successful completion
- supervise no more that four full-time or eight part-time doctoral students at one time, although the number can vary depending on other workload commitments.

Often a doctoral student has two supervisors, one familiar with the topic and one familiar with the research methodology. In some new university departments of nursing a supervisor who has not yet supervised doctoral students through to successful completion is mentored and advised by a senior colleague who meets all the above criteria. Thus some UK nurse doctoral students have two, or on rare occasions three, supervisors. In contrast a research group made up of several members may supervise an American doctoral student.

These process issues are explored in further detail by Holloway and Walker (2000). Doctoral students of nursing deserve to be taught by talented people who are prepared at doctoral level and who are themselves actively involved in generating and evaluating nursing knowledge and scholarship. Furthermore their research endeavours should be theoretically and philosophically relevant to the phenomena of specific interest to nurses and nursing. Whilst individual staff may have particular and diverse research interests, what would be more beneficial is a co-ordinated approach which still allows some room for individual flexibility within a larger, more focused and defined overall research strategy. Undertaking unrelated non-cumulative studies in a plethora of topics with no clear focus is not a good culture for a doctoral programme.

Normally for full-time students a supervisory session would take place one hour a week. For part-time students the average contact time is one hour a month. The student sends written work to the supervisor before the meeting so that issues can be discussed. Normally a detailed record is kept of the supervision meetings, indicating time of meeting, length of meeting, those present, preparation for the meeting, issues discussed and agreed and objectives, date and time for the next meeting.

Examination

The submitted thesis is sent to an external examiner who is an expert in the field and to an internal examiner who is a member of academic staff in the student's university. The examination of the thesis is based on broadly defined criteria which include the contribution to significant and original knowledge, that the work is worthy of publication in the public domain and that the candidate demonstrate in depth knowledge of the subject (UKCGE, 2002). The student defends the thesis to the examiners during a one- to two-hour oral examination (viva). Supervisors have observer status in the oral examination. Commonly there can be one of six outcomes to such an examination:

1. The student is awarded a PhD with no changes required to the thesis.
2. The student is awarded a PhD based on making minor changes to the thesis.
3. The student is awarded a PhD based on making more substantial changes to the thesis.
4. The student fails the PhD but is awarded a Master of Philosophy.
5. The student is awarded a Master of Philosophy based on making changes to the thesis.
6. The student fails the thesis outright.

After a successful defence at the viva, the relationship between the supervisor(s) and student continues with joint publications and conference presentations being the norm. In the UK a research assessment exercise audits the quality of a university's research infrastructure, activities and outputs. Within this scheme academic staff and university departments get credit for successful and timely PhD completions.

Postdoctoral careers

Doctoral study is best described as advanced scholarly training and the graduate represents an emergent scientist (Meleis, 1981). However, in order for doctorally prepared nurses to sharpen their skills to develop further the substantive knowledge base for nursing, they have to mature in a culture of postdoctoral scholarship and creativity. This realisation debunks the myth that once a doctorate degree is obtained the successful candidate can assume the role of an independent mature scientist and future research leader. Therefore it is imperative that doctoral graduates are encouraged to think about career development beyond the doctorate, and academic staff have a remit to guide and support them in the pursuit of postdoctoral study. A range of postdoctoral career pathways is required to facilitate exchange between practice and research (Wilson Barnett, 2001). Such opportunities for postdoctoral nurses and midwives ensure that skills are used in practice. In turn a strategy to develop research programmes within clinical areas would be provided and ultimately build much needed research and development capacity within the profession (Rafferty, 2000).

Conclusion

Doctorally prepared nurses have an obligation to current and future service users to search for new knowledge to underpin practice. In the UK the move to doctoral education for nurses has its dissenters. Our observations lead us to believe that these are mostly physicians or nurses who feel that nursing is moving too fast and is leaving behind or rejecting what they erroneously perceive to be important knowledge, skills and tasks. However, by definition, doctorally prepared nurses generate knowledge that makes a significant contribution to the discipline. This is the case whether the programme is a professional doctorate or a traditional PhD. This can only have positive implications for patient care.

It is evident that the historical development of doctoral study has differed internationally, reflecting varied health care and education systems, but also some similarities, such as movement of nursing into higher education and the relatively recent emergence of doctoral research, rapid development of new-style practice-focused programmes and the increase in part-time study. Therefore successful doctoral education seems to have several underpinning factors:

- the requirement for synergy between academic focus and practice issues
- the personal needs of students reflecting career trajectories with an increasing demand for continuing professional development in contrast to research training alone
- the widening professional base of higher education with increased vocational focus.

In current and future practice contexts post-doctoral nurses need a broad range of expertise, the ability to negotiate a diverse range of methods and research approaches, to be able to draw upon complex non-traditional data and to demonstrate expertise in critical reflection, supervision and leadership. These features provide a clear rationale for multiple doctorate programmes and pave the way for growth in a raft of new professional doctorate programmes.

Key points

- Generally the availability of doctoral programmes in nursing has increased, in addition new and diverse routes to doctoral preparation have emerged internationally.
- The mix of doctoral approaches is appropriate for the current stage of discipline development, with complementary roles of 'professional scholars' and 'scholarly professionals'.
- Post-doctoral nurses need a broad range of expertise and the ability to negotiate a diverse range of research approaches as well as to demonstrate critical reflection, supervision and leadership.
- Within practice disciplines such as nursing the core of doctoral study concerns the synergy between practice development, personal development and discipline development.

References

Anderson, C.A. (2000) Current Strengths and Limitations of Doctoral Education in Nursing; are we prepared for the future? *Journal of Professional Nursing*, **16**(4): 191–200.

Becher, T., Henkel, M. and Kogan, M. (1994) *Graduate Education in Britain*. London: Jessica Kingsley.

Benner, P. (1984) *From novice to expert. Excellence and Power in clinical nursing practice*. Menlo Park, CA: Addison Wesley.

Benoliel, J.Q. (1977) The interaction between theory and research. *Nursing Outlook*, **25**: 108–13.

Benz, V.M. and Shapiro, J.J. (1998) *Mindful Inquiry in Social Research*. Thousand Oaks: Sage.

Blancett, S.S. (1989) Defining doctoral education. *Nurse Educator*, **14**(3).

Boore, J.R.P. (1996) Postgraduate education in nursing: a case study. *Journal of Advanced Nursing*, **23**: 620–29.

Booth, C. (2001) Broader PhD courses start at 10 universities. *Research Fortnight*, 25th April. URL http://www.newphd.ac.uk

Bourner, T., Bowden, R. & Laing, S. (2001) Professional Doctorates in England. *Studies in Higher Education*, March, **26**(1): 65–94.

Doncaster, K. and Thorne, L. (2000). Reflection and Planning: essential elements of professional doctorates. *Reflective Practice*, **1**(3): 391–9.

Downs, F.S. (1978) Doctoral education in nursing: future directions. *Nursing Outlook*, **26**: 56–61.

Downs, F.S. (1988) Doctoral education: our claim to the future. *Nursing Outlook*, **36**: 18–20.

Downs, F. (1989) Differences between the professional doctorate and the academic/research doctorate. *Journal of Professional Nursing*, **5**: 261–5.

Galvin, K. and Carr, E. (2001) The emergence of professional doctorates: where are we and where are we going. Conference presentation, Bournemouth, UK.

Galvin, K.T. and Carr, E. (2003) the emergence of professional doctorates in nursing in the UK: where are we now? *Nursing Times Research*, **8**(4): 2–16.

Grace, H. (1978) The development of doctoral education in nursing: an historical perspective. *Journal of Nursing Education*, **17**: 17–27.

Guest, D., Redfern, S., Wilson-Barnett, J., Dewe, P., Peccei, R., Rosenthal, P., Evans, A., Young, C., Montgomery, J. & Oakley, P. (2001) *A Preliminary Evaluation of the Establishment of Nurse, Midwife and Health Visitor Consultants*: a report to the Department of Health. URL http://www.kcl.ac.uk/depsta/pse/mancen/ResearchPapers/NCP.htm

HEFCE (2000) *QAA Codes of Practice*. Bristol: HEFCE.

HESA (Higher Education Statistics Agency) (1999) *Students in Higher Education Institutions 1997/1998*. Cheltenham: HESA.

Holloway, I. and Walker, J. (2000) *Getting a PhD in Health and Social Care*. Oxford: Blackwell Science.

Hudacek, S. and Carpenter, D.R. (1998) Student perceptions of nurse doctorates: Similarities and Differences. *Journal of Professional Nursing,* **14**(1): 14–21.

INDEN (International Network of Doctoral Education) (2002) *Quality Criteria and Indicators of Doctoral Education* (QCI). URL http://www.umich.edu/~inden/

Ketefian, S., Neves, E.P. and Gutierrez, M.G. (2001) Nursing Doctorate education in the Americas. *Online Journal of Issues in Nursing,* **5**(2): 8.

Lanara, V.A. (1994) The contribution of nursing research to the development of the discipline of nursing in Europe. Proceedings from the 7th Biennial Conference, Oslo: Workgroup of European Nurse Researchers.

Lancaster, L.E. (1984) Doctoral Education in Nursing, the Sisyphian Concept, and Pandora's Box. Guest Editorial, *Critical Care Nurse,* **4**(3): 6–17.

Lash, A.A. (1987) Rival conceptions in doctoral education in nursing and their outcomes: an update. *Journal of Nursing Education,* **26**: 221–66.

Mason, C. and McKenna, H.P. (1995) How to survive a Ph.D. *Nurse Researcher,* **2**(3): 73–9.

McKenna, H.P. and Cutcliffe, J. (2001) Nursing doctorate education in the United Kingdom and Ireland. *Online Journal of Issues in Nursing,* **5**: 2–9.

Meleis, A.I. (1981) Nursing Theory and scholarliness in the doctoral programme. *Advances in Nursing Science,* **3**: 31–41.

Newman, M. (1975) The professional Doctorate in nursing: Position paper. *Nursing Outlook,* **23**: 704–6.

Polanyi, M. (1958) *Personal Knowledge.* Chicago: University of Chicago Press.

Quality Assurance Agency for Higher Education (1999) Postgraduate research programme. Codes of practice quality and standards in HE. www.qaa.ac.uk/public/cop/cop/contents.htm

Rafferty, A.M. (2000) *Influencing the research and development agenda.* Paper presented to a Department of Health R&D workshop, York, March.

Seitz, P. (1987) The pros and cons of doctoral education. *The Canadian Nurse,* **83**(5): 27.

Towell, D. (1975) Understanding Psychiatric Nursing: A sociological study of modern psychiatric nursing practice. London: Royal College of Nursing.

Traynor, M. (1997) Personal communication.

Traynor, M. and Rafferty, A.M. (1998) *Nursing Research and the Higher Education Context. A second working paper.* London: Centre for Policy in Nursing Research, London School of Hygiene and Tropical Medicine.

UK Council for Graduate Education (UKCGE) (1996) *Practice Based Doctorates in Creative and Peforming Arts and Design.* Warwick: UKCGE.

UK Council for Graduate Education (UKCGE) (1998) *The Status of Published Work in Submissions for Doctoral Degrees in European Universities*. Warwick: UKCGE.

UK Council for Graduate Education (UKCGE) (2002) Professional Doctorates. Warwick: UKCGE.

West, K.M. (1966) The case against teaching. *Journal of Medical Education*, **41**: 766–71.

Wilson Barnett (2001) Editorial Research Capacity in Nursing. *International Journal of Nursing Studies*, **38**(3): 241–2.

Ziemer, M., Brown, J., Fitzpatrick, M.L., Manfriedi, C., O'Leary, J. and Valiga, T.M. (1992) Doctoral programmes in nursing: philosophy, curricula, and programme requirements. *Journal of Professional Nursing*, **8**: 56–62.

7 Introduction to careers in nursing research: Case studies and opportunities

Veronica Bishop

I knew who I was this morning but I've changed a few times since then.
Lewis Carroll (1982)

This chapter discusses various options and opportunities for a career in nursing research and illustrates examples with case studies. Drawing together the strands held in common by each case history it is apparent that each had an openness to multidisciplinary working and to the involvement of peer review from other disciplines as well as their own. This allows for a breadth of knowledge and influence complementary to nursing and to its future as a mature profession.

Introduction

There is substantial evidence being collected as I write that researcher practitioner roles are developing, bringing with them new opportunities to practice research-based care in the health services. Indeed a recent study by Bryar (2003) found that the required skills for undertaking research are accumulating considerably. This is good news for the global initiative of developing research capacity in health care and good, too, for the individual who really wants to provide the best possible care based on sound evidence. However, as Bryar notes, the subsequent utilisation of these skills results from the practitioner's own motivation rather than being a requirement of subsequent posts.

In this chapter the profiles of five motivated nurses, active in research and striving to connect clinical practice with research and development, each in their own unique way, are presented. These are of particular relevance to readers who are considering the opportunities to 'break into' research and how they might build on existing models. Remember, nothing is cast in stone. Roles and careers are very dynamic, reflecting the needs and economic pressures of the day. In reading this chapter it is not necessary to know the people, nor those who mentored them during their careers. What is important is to draw out those issues which are common to each, and to reflect on how to make your way in your career.

Having a career in research in any discipline is often perceived as rather rarefied and those people involved as not being of the real world, a notion exacerbated by the media, particularly films who stereotypically portray anyone doing research as a boffin and slightly crazy. Unfortunately these very limited perceptions pertain as much to nursing as to any other field and do no service to the profession. Career pathways in research can take one of several turns. I began my research career as a member of a multi-disciplinary team involved in pharmacological studies, gaining valuable experience and grasping the opportunity presented to work for higher degrees. Being a research assistant is often the first step in a research career, leading to opportunities to become a research fellow, then possibly a senior fellow. This progressive pathway leads to skills gained in developing grant applications for funding, writing protocols and reports and getting published in peer review journals as a collaborative and single author. This is the development of a personal portfolio, as discussed in Chapter 8. It is vital throughout this development, and for all your professional life, to keep an up-to-date record of every paper presented, every paper published – these are vital components of your curriculum vitae (CV) and as time passes it is alarming how difficult it is to remember all your activities. Your CV is your passport to greater challenges and, hopefully, rewards both mental and monetary. It is also important to know the differences between levels of appointments and the concomitant expectations if you are to avoid setting yourself up to fail or, conversely, not being adventurous enough for your expertise when applying for research posts. Kenkre and Foxcroft (2001) highlight typical advertisements for different posts, a practical exercise for anyone considering a new career pathway.

Having discussed the first steps in a career in research it is useful to consider where such journeys may lead. The profiles of nurses who currently hold key roles in nursing research are presented here to illustrate that, while each person is highly individual, each is truly part of the professional whole and moves with dedicated commitment to maintaining that professional unity. This unity does not imply an uncritical, sycophantic allegiance to a single methodology for nursing research; indeed the case against this is well made in Chapter 4 where Freshwater examines differing paradigms and highlights the ongoing debates. If nursing does not enter into debate and does not question itself it is unlikely to have much to contribute to the larger agenda of health care and should not be called a profession.

These individuals range from well-established to new in the field, and each has pursued diverse paths, thus affording the reader an insight into many options. The voices of the writers come though clearly, and I have not sought to change or interfere with their very individual styles of writing, as that would destroy their 'colour'. What I have done is to draw out key indicators and highlighted these in the Conclusion, which may be helpful for those seeking career advice, particularly (but not necessarily) in research into health care.

Case study 1.   Ann McMahon, Director, RCN Research and Development Centre, Manchester University

Never doubt that a small group of thoughtful, committed citizens can change the world; indeed, it's the only thing that ever has. Margaret Mead (1901–78) (Attrib).

Introduction

I went to Dundee College of Technology (now University of Abertay) to undertake a degree in nursing after a false start studying for a biochemistry degree at St Andrews University. The biochemistry degree at the prestigious university was what I felt was expected of me. The nursing degree at the local college of technology was what I knew in my heart I wanted to do. I elected to register in both general and mental health nursing largely as a result of the inspirational leadership of the course director, an eminent psychiatric nurse academic. Much of the teaching

I received was evidence based and the majority of my lecturers were undertaking a degree or a higher degree themselves. I met many inspirational teachers and leaders during my undergraduate studies but the one who will always stand out for me was the stoma therapist. I was overwhelmed by the richness of her knowledge, grounded in her day-to-day practice and the subsequent quality of her teaching.

I graduated in 1983 aspiring to become a clinical nurse specialist in the fulness of time. I staffed on an acute male surgical ward and while there I began to realise that I was particularly interested in supporting patients through the psychological impact of physical illness. I began to question whether I was able to give the level of support I felt was required within that environment.

First steps on the research journey

I moved to Manchester in 1984 and took up post as a staff nurse on the acute medical oncology unit at the Christie Hospital – very busy! But the culture very much focused on the physical *and* psychological well-being of both patients and their families/ partners. Here I met a nurse who spent time on our ward as part of the clinical component of her Masters degree in Nursing at Manchester University. I enjoyed talking to her about her course and her research. After nearly two years as a staff nurse I took up post as a clinical nurse specialist in intravenous chemotherapy. In this role I met with my colleague who had completed her Masters degree and was undertaking a PhD. She invited me to take part in her pilot study looking at nurses' communications skills. I tape-recorded encounters with patients and was given feedback and coaching on my communications skills. This was a worthwhile experience that really helped me to see the potential of nursing research within a clinical setting.

There was a very strong research culture, particularly in the medical oncology team, and I was made to feel very much a part of the research endeavour and was asked to write elements of research protocols where nursing care was imperative to the research process. This led to extensive networking with nursing colleagues and recognition through authorship of protocols and publications. Through the combination of being a part of that culture and working with my PhD student colleague I began to realise that 'nurses were doing it for themselves'. I therefore applied for a place on the Masters programme at Manchester University. My vision was to remain in clinical practice and do so with a Masters degree – this was almost unheard of then. Almost all of the other students in my cohort were nurse teachers and lecturers and they were funded by the English National Board (ENB) to undertake the course. I was turned down for ENB funding at interview because I didn't want to leave clinical practice and work within a school of nursing teaching pre-registration nurses. I would have been happy teaching within my specialty – cancer nursing – in a joint appointment role, but that was not an option then. I received support from the Director of Nursing who found resources to assist me, including a 12-month secondment so that afterwards I could return to my post. I managed to secure additional financial help to enable me to support myself throughout the year.

Significant decisions along the way

During the Masters programme we had a session to talk about the research we were interested in, to match students with potential supervisors. I was interested in the problem of anticipatory nausea and vomiting in patients receiving chemotherapy and stated that I had heard of several interventions to manage this symptom, including behavioural therapy. One of the departmental professors with a background in mental health immediately saw the connection with nurses working in advanced mental health practice and my interest. He put me in contact with two nurse behavioural therapists who trained me in progressive muscle relaxation (PMR) and cognitive therapy. This became the intervention that I used in my research. Undertaking a Masters degree, within an academic environment and with a very proactive supervisor, encouraged me to disseminate my research.

I returned to work, inspired by my year out and ready to put my new research skills into practice. However my sponsor, the Director of Nursing Services (DNS) had gone on maternity leave. It felt as though the organisation neither valued nor knew now what to do with my skills. Indeed at worst I was left with the impression that I was perceived as a threat. I found myself at a crossroads. My supervisor was hoping that he could create a post within the university suited to me. At the same time I was advised of an advertisement for an assistant director of nursing services leading on research and development (R&D) within a district general hospital. What was I to do? I decided that I didn't have a real dilemma unless I applied for the job and was offered it. To my total amazement the theoretical dilemma became a very real one. After a great deal of soul-searching I decided to take the lead R&D role because I felt that in that one I would have more influence. I think the DNS who appointed me took a risk as I had no people management experience and this job was about managing both projects and managing a team. As the role developed I took the lead within the organisation in translating national health and social care policy to make sense of it in practice. It involved a rich mix of policy development, quality improvement work, informatics, practice development, research and evaluation. Whilst in that role a colleague and I lobbied the then director of policy and practice at the Royal College of Nursing (RCN). We felt that there was a lack of leadership in nursing. The director set up a small group and our thinking resulted in the RCN's clinical leadership programme. This was the closest I had become to taking on an activist role at the RCN.

It was during the Thatcher Years that the NHS began to embrace managerialism. This no doubt had some benefits, such as a strong focus on service quality. However, in my view efficiency drives at times militated against delivering a quality service. How could I lead on quality improvement and development when the workforce was being pared to the quick and morale was at an all-time low? I thought, perhaps naively, that the solution was to seek out a director of nursing post for myself and defend nursing establishments from a board position.

As I was looking, my current post at the RCN was advertised as research adviser. I decided the opportunity to work for my professional organisation was a once in lifetime opportunity and was delighted to get the job, which I took up in 1994. In this post I have mapped out and implemented the RCN's R&D Strategy, which has included the establishment of the RCN's R&D co-ordinating centre and a programme of work on research commissioning, infrastructure and dissemination. None of this would have been possible without the fantastic opportunity to work with some of the brightest and most committed members of the profession and an amazingly supportive team. During this time I have also undertaken a three-year taught MPhil in critical management at Lancaster University, which has been profoundly challenging. I converted my MPhil to a PhD dissertation in 2001.

Next steps

Currently I am working with a group of experts to promote excellence in R&D in NHS trusts and project managing and agenda to manage nursing knowledge more effectively across the RCN. In my PhD dissertation I am examining innovations in service delivery from a critical perspective.

I now believe that there are multiple ways to influence agendas and that rising up the career ladder is only one way. I am working hard to develop and refine my writing skills and am extremely grateful for the encouragement and support I have received from my critical friends who help me along the way.

Case study 2.   Steven Ersser, Head of Nursing Development, School of Nursing and Midwifery, University of Southampton

> Afoot and light-hearted I take the open road,
> Healthy, free, the world before me,
> The long brown path before me leading wherever I choose.
>
> Walt Whitman (1871)

Introduction

My introduction to nursing came originally from childhood when my mother, who was an ardent first-aid activist, constantly handed me the manual asking me to test her on the theory and practice. Given that we lived near a major London road where accidents were frequent, this was not a mere academic pastime. In the intervening years I was a patient for a prolonged period, taking most of my A levels in hospital. Convinced that I wanted to be involved in health care and determined to study at university level I was less clear as to the route I wished to follow. The stereotypical doctor role did not feel comfortable to me, but I was unaware that nursing could then be studied at degree level. As a patient I gained some insight into the scope and impact of good nursing. It was subsequently a great discovery for me that it was possible to combine university life with nurse training, so this is the path I chose.

First steps of the research journey

The initial stimulus to improve nursing care through research came during my time as an undergraduate nursing student in London. From this point onwards I was fortunate to have research teaching from nurses who were to become leaders in the profession. Both of these dynamic professionals were strong advocates for research on nursing and for the need to maintain a critical view of the profession that is offered by the social sciences. I left higher education with an idealistic aspiration to combine professional development with the ability to examine its rhetoric and practices. After gaining clinical experience in London I took my first of many divergent career steps by working at the Oxford Nursing Development Unit (ONDU). I arrived in Oxford, where I was to remain for 13 years, at a time of significant experimentation within nursing. The unit's leaders welcomed the opportunity to explore and test clinical developments through clinical work, review and research investigation. This formative period in my career helped me to retain a focus on research. This stimulating setting became the impetus for my registering part time for a research degree; the study examined assumptions on the therapeutic nature and impact of nursing.

My next major step was to the National Institute of Nursing, a new type of academic centre that set out to investigate nursing practice development in a systematic way. The directors valued the need to study nursing by retaining a close proximity to practice as well as sometimes cultivating distance. I started as a research student and then became a research fellow. Subsequently I moved into one of the new lecturer–practitioner posts as an

Institute employee, combining my work leading nursing in a dermatology department with teaching and research. I received valued mentorship from my academic medical colleagues which continues to this day. Within my research role I continued to undertake my doctorate and studied the process of developmental change with Institute colleagues. However, the lecturer–practitioner roles were unduly complex in the early stages. As a researcher I felt a degree of frustration in advancing my studies, given the demands of my role.

At the same time I was a part-time research student at King's College, London. King's offered me a sufficient degree of detachment that was necessary to further my studies. I see now that it was necessary to have more protected time to complete my doctoral thesis. At King's I greatly benefited from another intellectual community and the opportunity to exchange with another strong group of researchers and research students; this helped to reduce the isolation research students sometimes feel. Mentorship again became key, not only from my supervisors within Kings but also from my associate supervisor back in Oxford. This was perhaps particularly helpful as this mentor provided insight as a sociologist, thus assisting me to cultivate a more detached view of nursing.

Significant decisions along the way

When my secondment to practice ended as a lecturer–practitioner at both the Institute and Oxford Polytechnic (now Oxford Brookes University) I decided to move into full-time higher education to lead a new advanced practice master's course and to help set up the Oxford Centre for Health Care Research & Development. The Centre was a valuable stimulus in its multi-professional research environment and opportunities for external collaboration with other health sciences centres in Oxford. I had completed my PhD and now helped to develop a research infrastructure for others as well as myself.

Although by this stage relatively senior in nursing terms, I was a new post-doctoral researcher. Looking back, the level of responsibility undertaken by such researchers in nursing compared with 'post-docs' in other fields is surprising. Today this is less likely because there are more suitable staff around. In an ideal world I would have tried harder to plan my own post-doctoral programme of work earlier. I continued to work on my clinical interest area, dermatology and skin care, which struck me as a fascinating but greatly neglected area of study. During this period I received significant support from my colleagues, although there were limited opportunities for me to find the right research mentorship. I was appointed as a senior research fellow and then later as Reader in Nursing.

I felt by this time that I needed time to step out and away from the city I had worked in for many years and reflected on what might be the next steps in my career. This came through an invitation to apply as a visiting scholar to St John's College, Cambridge. A fellow who was both a sociologist and a key figure in the Psoriasis Association made this possible. He recognised my wish to develop the study of skin care and dermatology and to consolidate my work. This rare offer came just at the right time. It made a considerable difference to have a period to stand back, to be relieved of most work responsibilities, to debate and to refocus. It was refreshing to be exposed to an environment of researchers in which the nursing and health care research was novel (the only other nursing connection I could find was Lady Margaret Beaufort, the College's foundress of 1511). To explain the research questions and their investigation to those who were so detached from nursing was valuable. I then spent part of the summer at the John Hartford Institute of Geriatric Nursing at New York University. I gained insight into a well-organised and well-resourced research centre in the USA. The wider horizons and mentorship opportunities received during this sabbatical period where invaluable. I returned from my sabbatical ready for a new work setting. I sought an academic setting where there was an established research culture and an aspiration to build a strong research focus for nursing, and strong practice links. I was appointed as Head of Nursing Development at the University of Southampton, School of Nursing & Midwifery, where I remain today. My role is essentially as one of a group of research leads. There is much to be gained from being in a faculty of medicine, an environment that fosters cross-links with other clinical disciplines. My position at Southampton allowed me to start to build a team in my research focus area, the behavioural and biological basis of skin vulnerability. Although these are still early days we have a group, not only researchers but also of development and clinical staff, who are involved in the field of skin care. I am fortunate to work with a number of talented researchers. I continue to benefit from the mentorship on offer from my peers and senior colleagues. The challenge is now, more than ever before, to work effectively as a scientific group to address complex research issues. A significant part of my role is to provide guidance to others.

Next steps

It is in the nature of people's career paths, as with all paths in life, that they are largely unpredictable and, certainly in the case of my research career, a long and winding road. I really do wonder if I can say that I have had a 'research career'. Undoubtedly I have had a continuous research career *strand* throughout my *nursing* career, but this has been interwoven with co-existent roles as a practitioner, teacher and manager. Taking opportunities to learn from the interface between practice, research and education has been a feature of my career path. Other features include the support and teaching I have received from others and, to be candid, an element of being in the right place at the right time.

Summing up during my career so far. I maintained a strand of research that has grown in activity, although I continue to move across the different elements of my role and try to take advantage of their synergy. I continue to try to work closely with the practice setting and health service at its different levels. I retain a belief in the importance of finding the right mix of involvement and detachment to study nursing effectively. My next goals are to continue to strengthen my links and exchanges with social and biological scientists, as well as clinicians in my field, both here and abroad. Trying to integrate the various strands of one's role as a leader in research and development and to question and demonstrate positive change in practice remains the constant challenge. As time goes by I wish to spend more time encouraging and challenging others, feeling that in the past I have had more than my fair share of encouragement and challenge from many outstanding individuals both inside and outside of nursing. These people have generously shared their time and talents; there has been no greater assistance along my career path than this.

Case study 3.   Sabi Redwood, Senior Lecturer in Research, IHCS, Bournemouth University

The moral quest for the good life and right action lies beyond the quest for knowledge alone. It requires passionate action guided by intelligent thought. (Garrison, 1997, summing up Dewey's stance towards moral practice)

Introduction

I couldn't say for certain that research did not feature in my pre-registration nurse training, but I don't remember leaving the school of nursing with any understanding about its role in my professional life. Furthermore it did not answer the questions I was beginning to ask as a new staff nurse. How do you hold and comfort a child who has been abused? How do you communicate with a mother whose baby is dying of AIDS and whose language you do not speak? How do you touch and move the lifeless and flaccid limbs belonging to an adolescent who is mourning the loss of their function? The scientific method of reducing and measuring to which I had been introduced offered little promise in helping me tackle these human concerns. I began to ask these questions of my elders and betters who quickly pointed me to more education to pacify me. Then one day I sat in a classroom and the tutor presented me with a completely new way of looking at the world. It felt as if I was the only student sitting in this classroom as she led my discovery of ways to answering my questions. A recent rummage through dusty cases in my loft produced the essays I wrote at that time: pieces in which I riled against Descartes, vilified quantitative research and heaped scorn on a science which neglected the human condition and impoverished nursing while I praised the extraordinary value of Kath Melia's and Janice Morse's work. However, my passion for qualitative research cooled as I tried to balance the needs of my young family with the demands of clinical practice and professional ambition. I was still relatively young when I reached what I had thought of as the pinnacle of my career: the post of senior sister of four children's wards. The talk was of budgets, efficiency savings and clinical effectiveness; my daily bread consisted of ensuring there were enough staff to cover the wards.

There were unreasonable expectations from the powers above and unreasonable demands from the nursing staff. After some years I realised that the cost to me as a person was too great and I looked for ways to re-invent myself professionally.

First steps on the research journey

An opportunity arose for a six-month secondment to do a piece of research for the hospital trust which employed me around the topic of patients' perceptions of personal care and how well it was being done. I grasped the opportunity to do this project, choosing to use grounded theory methodology and to get to know colleagues from the university who would later be instrumental in supporting my development as a researcher. My interest in the exploration of learning in practice was awakened when, during the data collection phase of this first project, I witnessed an ordinary, everyday interaction between a nurse and a patient.

I observed a young nurse sitting by the bed of an elderly woman, giving her water to drink through a feeder cup. The patient's face was gaunt and had a yellow tinge, and her breathing rattled noisily. The process of feeding was slow and laborious, as the woman could not hold much water in her mouth; much of it dribbled down her chin which the nurse carefully mopped up. At first she was awkward in holding the feeder cup and in positioning herself and her patient. She had also not yet developed a sense for how much water the woman was able to swallow at one time, and she did not allow the patient to catch her breath after swallowing and breathe for a while after the effort of it. Once the patient choked and struggled to cough. I could not see her face, but I could see the nurse's body tense in anxiety as the patient fought to clear her throat. She looked at her helplessly, murmuring apologies, and then hesitantly reached for the suction apparatus connected to the wall. However, after a few moments the coughing subsided without any intervention. The nurse then repositioned herself and slightly moved the patient's head. This small adjustment made feeding her patient much easier. She then learned to go with the patient's rhythm of breathing through the mouth, sipping a little water, breathing through the nose and swallowing, followed by a moment's rest. Not too long to tire her patient, nor too short to rush her. I saw the nurse relax her body and develop an ease as she was slowly feeding her patient. She then began to speak slowly to the woman who responded by opening her eyes and looking at her. They spoke little, but for some time both women were in an intimate dialogue with each other.

As I left the ward I felt myself to be very fortunate. I realised that I had just witnessed a new member of our profession learn the highly complex and deeply human skill of enabling another to drink. What I had seen was Nursing. And I began to ask questions again. How did she learn the skill of feeding a patient who struggled to breathe? What happened between her and the woman that enabled her to learn from her? I already had a sense that the challenge of answering those questions was going to be to render visible that which is essentially private experience and to lay it open in such a way that others may both see and understand some aspects of its meaning. 'Meaning' in this enterprise would have to move beyond cognitive and intellectual understanding, but to speak to something intuitive and practical within those seeking answers to similar questions. I also began to realise that the challenge of bringing that which is hidden to light is a methodological one; representing what has been brought to light would be a profoundly political one. I was beginning to grapple with the issues which were going to exercise me in the future.

Significant decisions along the way

Following the successful completion of my first research project I was very fortunate to be given the opportunity to lead several practice education research projects. I owe much to those who believed in me and supported me in developing my new skills both in researching and in managing research. I also discovered that far from being irrelevant, my previous experience as senior sister had equipped me well for my new job. I had learned to plan processes, negotiate barriers, solve problems and, crucially, to listen.

At the time I was also studying for a Master of Arts degree, an experience which, like the one some years earlier, opened up for me new ways of thinking and looking at world. The course enabled me to meet other students and academics who introduced me to concepts and ideas which sparked off my own imagination and creativity while at the same time sustaining a part of me that had lain unexamined. That part yearned to find out more about the world and about how people in the human service professions learned. I felt a strong desire to participate in the creation of knowledge and to 'do research'. But the research I wanted to do had to always be 'for' something, not be an end in itself: research for improvement, for bringing about a practical engagement, for action.

Next steps

Research for me cannot be something that produces reports gathering dust on a shelf. It has to speak to people, and I see it as my task to involve those who would be my audience, who should not be passive recipients, but engaged and immersed activists. I find this desire reflected in John Dewey's work, and while I still have far to travel in my career in nursing research this quote will always guide my work: 'The moral quest for the good life and right action lies beyond the quest for knowledge alone. It requires passionate action guided by intelligent thought.'

Case study 4.   Brendan McCormack, Professor of Nursing Research/Director of Nursing Research and Practice Development between the University of Ulster and the Royal Hospitals Trust, Belfast

> The reasonable man [sic] adapts himself to the world; the unreasonable man persists in trying to adapt the world to himself. Therefore, all progress depends on the unreasonable man. George Bernard Shaw (1903)

Introduction

I have chosen to begin this reflection with a quotation from George Bernard Shaw (one of the few heroes I admit to having in my life). When I read this quotation in a collected works of Shaw it resonated with my experience of being a nurse and brought clarity concerning decisions I have made about my career and the choices that I have made. Key to this reflection is the notion of being 'unreasonable' and the idea that progress is dependent on unreasonableness.

I began nursing in 1980 more by chance than plan. My subjects in school focused on me pursuing a career in plastics engineering, something I knew I didn't want to do. Having failed one of the key subjects I needed to get to university (technical drawing) the decision was made for me and I found myself open to a range of career options and very excited by this. The local psychiatric hospital where I lived in Ireland advertised for student nurses and for reasons unknown to me I applied and was offered a place. It was not the most popular decision I made in my life, and members of my family actively discouraged me from accepting the place (there is no history of nursing or health care in my family tree). It is true to say that my experience as a psychiatric nurse has shaped everything I have done since. I had to grow up very quickly to survive and, while I knew I did not want to be a psychiatric nurse, I did know that I enjoyed nursing. My reflection on the impact of my psychiatric nursing experience has been published elsewhere. Four months after qualifying as an RMN I secured a place in England to undertake an 18-month post-registration training as a general nurse. Despite ritualistic, routinised and hierarchical practices, I loved every moment of it and knew I had made a good decision.

First steps of the research journey

Soon after securing my first staff nurse position I began a diploma in professional studies in nursing (DPSN), and that set the ball rolling for a career in research and practice development. My first staff nurse position as an RGN was in trauma orthopaedics. The senior nurse manager of the orthopaedic unit suggested within the first month of my appointment that I should apply to undertake a diploma in professional studies in nursing and facilitated me doing so. It was during this course that my insight into nursing and its potential really began. It was my first introduction to research-based knowledge and theoretical perspectives. It was like a whole new world opening up in front of me, and despite the hassle of part-time study it was a fantastic experience. Whilst some of the course work was difficult, frustrating and at times appeared irrelevant, the support of fellow course colleagues and facilitators made the experience worthwhile. Of most significance is one particular experience. I had not written an academic essay since leaving school as all of my nursing courses were assessed using multiple-choice examinations. My first assignment on Florence Nightingale was of a very poor standard. The course leader recognised this and provided one-to-one tuition in essay writing. This support helped me to learn to read research critically and engage in critical thinking. This way of thinking became an everyday part of my practice and undertaking further study reflected an increasing desire to critically question my practice and that of others. I transferred my diploma into a degree in nursing, and soon after I completed a post graduate certificate in adult education (PGCEA) and, while doing this, got my biggest and luckiest break in that I was appointed as clinical lecturer in nursing in Oxford. The position came with a scholarship to undertake a doctorate in philosophy at the University of Oxford.

Significant decisions

Throughout this time I created a number of joint appointment roles that enabled me to stay in clinical practice, teach and undertake practice development and research. My move to Oxford acted as a catalyst for this, being formalised in the positions I held and my doctoral studies. I had always been interested in older people and practice development and the roles I held enabled me to develop expertise in both. Returning to the 'unreasonable man', my experience as a psychiatric nurse became a key focus of my doctoral studies. I was studying the issue of 'the autonomy of older people in hospital' utilising a hermeneutic approach. The nature of hermeneutics requires the engagement of the self of the researcher with the research topic. It became very clear that my experiences as a psychiatric nurse had shaped my passion for developing practice. Shaw argues that progress only happens when people behave unreasonably. I interpret that as meaning, not accepting the status quo, asking critical questions and challenging 'prevailing norms'. I realised in the course of this work that this desire was driven by my experiences of institutionalisation. This understanding significantly shaped my research work and my subsequent practice development activity. The clarity that ensued enabled me to see the importance of practice development shaped in a research context. Since then I have been undertaking systematic practice development research, with an emphasis on demonstrating the importance of systematic approaches to practice development and the advancement of knowledge in this field ... and of course a major emphasis on services for older people. I have had key mentors and role models who have helped me with this work and I believe that it was through their mentorship and critical companionship that I have been able to operationalise my current role. In addition, studying at the University of Oxford exposed me to a way of thinking that I had not previously encountered and to some of the great philosophers and lead philosophical thinkers. This experience was invaluable in shaping my understanding of research, appreciating the importance of philosophy and learning how to engage in critical debate.

Next steps

At the outset I have to come clean and say that few of my career decisions were initiated by me, as for many years I lacked confidence in my abilities. Instead many wonderful mentors, managers and role models encouraged, enthused and initiated career changes on my behalf. I am extremely grateful to these people. I was contacted by a recruitment firm and asked to apply for the post that I currently occupy. I had never considered myself to be professor material and was a bit overwhelmed by the idea of holding such a position. Competing for and being successful in securing this position has helped to eliminate the lack of confidence that has haunted my career. But, more importantly, the organisation of the role, with a formal position in an NHS trust, has meant that my continued (but more measured) passion for nursing practice research and development is legitimised. Colleagues regularly challenge the legitimacy of the research approaches I adopt in terms of their scientific basis (that is, 'is practitioner research and practice development really research?'). However, my previous experiences, the mentors and role models who have helped me and my ability to systematically reflect on my effectiveness means that I am very comfortable in defending these research approaches. I am proud to be in a professorial position that is located in clinical practice and even more proud to be seen as a practice developer and practitioner researcher – the pinnacle of 'unreasonableness'! Our socialisation as nurses is a key part of the way we make choices in our practice and in our career progression. It is only recently that I have managed to identify a pattern to my career choices and more importantly the significance of my early nursing experiences in these choices. For me, being an effective researcher requires systematic reflection, but systematic reflection requires self-awareness and engagement in our reality. My practice development mantra of 'understanding the past in order to work in the present and create a future' seems equally important to understanding our careers.

Case study 5.   Dawn Freshwater, Professor of Mental Health and Primary Care and Lead for Academic Centre in Practice, IHCS, Bournemouth University and North/South West Dorset NHS Trusts

> When you think of things, you find sometimes that a thing which seemed very thingish inside you is quite different when it gets out into the open and has other people looking at it. (Pooh bear, 2002)

Introduction

I knew I wanted to be a nurse before I left school and had a place when I was 16, so I decided to earn some money for a while while waiting for my 18th birthday to arrive. I worked in an estate agent's where I learnt about working with people in high-stress situations. I operated the switchboard and was often on the receiving end of some nasty comments, unsuitable for publication here. Now, as I look back on that time, I realise I was conducting my own heuristic research, testing out through trial and error ways of keeping myself and others calm and rational in what were often emotionally charged circumstances.

I had sat the GNC entrance test to secure my place as a student nurse and had to work extremely hard to ensure that I kept it. It never occurred to me that I would follow a career pathway that would lead me into the academy and into research. My main aim was to become a staff nurse and work on the wards. This I did, practising in acute settings for several years before becoming a sister and eventually moving out into the community to become a practice nurse. It was this move that provided me with my first real opportunity to be involved in clinical research, this and my decision to enter higher education, which also opened many doors for me.

First steps on the research journey

I was undertaking an ENB course in practice nursing (this was before the era of nurse practitioners in the UK) and was involved in a small scale profiling project based in the practice where I was based. One of the GP's approached me to ask if I would like to be involved in a national research project. It was in the late 1980s and the Royal London Hospital was leading the national screening programme for ovarian cancer. The discovery that early intervention might save the lives of women at risk from ovarian cancer had led to the development of national centres at which eligible women could be screened. I took the lead on this project within the practice and became committed to making it work at a local level. The national project was very successful and I was delighted to attend a fundraising and appreciation event at the Merchant Taylor's Hall in London alongside many other nurses, researchers, general practitioners and celebrities. Indeed my claim to fame has been that I lunched with Piers Brosnan, later to become 007.

Around the same time I was undertaking modules in research and research methods as part of my degree in nursing with the Royal College of Nursing. I had never really considered myself bright and was surprised to find that I was managing the coursework on the degree reasonably well providing I continued to work at it. I was even more surprised to discover that I was achieving nearly top marks in the research modules (unlike some of the other modules) without finding it too hard going. I am sure this was not down to my intellectual grasp of the research methods but was essentially driven by my nosiness, curiosity and an interesting research topic. And by this I mean one that was personally meaningful. I delighted in the research literature and found writing my research proposal an absolute joy, I became completely immersed in it.

This enthusiasm continued into my dissertation, which overtook me – I found myself surrounded by questionnaires, books and other reading materials, and half-analysed data. I was really enjoying it, but found it frustrating having to leave it to engage in other areas of my learning and practice. It often appeared to me that my learning and practice were treated as if they were separate from the research that I was carrying out, fragmenting me along with my practice. Research was, of course, also changing my view of practice. At this time I was involved in teaching as well as maintaining a clinical practice and I soon recognised the impact of the shift in my thinking and questioning. After I had finished my dissertation my supervisor and I realised that I had 'the bug' – or rather the bug had me. I became increasingly involved in teaching about research methods to my colleagues in the community and was also encouraged to do some teaching at the school of nursing, where the ENB research course was just being set up.

Significant decisions along the way

Almost immediately after completing my first degree I registered for an MPhil with Nottingham University; although, on reflection, I had little idea of what I was letting myself in for. My intention was to complete an MPhil; it was really at the suggestion of my supervisor that I considered upgrading to a PhD. Doing a PhD part time and working full was an experience that really put my commitment and stamina to the test. During this time I was also converting my previous experience as a counsellor into a registrable qualification with the United Kingdom Council for Psychotherapists. My experiences of research at first-degree level and subsequently at higher-degree level were of course completely different. Learning the rather idealistic theories and methods of research for health care and then working with them in dynamic, chaotic and often uncertain practice settings was a challenge that

I hadn't bargained for. This was where I learnt that the transferable skills and adaptability I had gained as a practising nurse were fundamental to the local and contingent application of research theories, methods and practices.

I have always been an avid reader and have fond memories of reading and re-reading the same books over and over again when I was young. One that springs to mind is *The Tales of Hans Christian Andersen*. I guess there has always been something about stories that captivates me, getting caught up in the tale that is not only being told but also being invented as it is told. I realise now that this links to my passion for qualitative research and in particular narrative and reflexivity. My love of stories has been one of the motivating factors in directing me to a deep interest in reflective practice and of course my own biography.

Such was my interest in research and its relevance to practice that I took up a fixed-term appointment as senior research fellow knowing that the funding was not long term. This post enabled me to work across many disciplines and to develop a clear programme of work, which was of use to both the university and the hospitals to which I was responsible. By this time I had been writing for publication and found that this was something that I also enjoyed, particularly disseminating research findings in creative and challenging ways and, more latterly, raising questions about the utility of research within health care. Thus my love of stories somehow turned into a desire to write my own. This was one of the biggest surprises, as I was really not sure I had anything of any value to say. On reflection I realise that writing is not just about what you have to say, it is also a process of learning.

The opportunity to write with others always provides a chance to learn about oneself in many ways if one is prepared to make oneself vulnerable to the constructive criticism of others. This is of course essential to a successful research career, not least in relation to seeking funding and proposal writing, many of which I have had rejected. My joint appointment gave me the opportunity to really concentrate my efforts on developing a research career. I was able to work collaboratively with others, both nationally and internationally, and to identify areas of concern for nurses, nursing care, nurse education and indeed other disciplines.

Next steps

Many experiences have contributed to the development of my career in nursing, some more notable than others. People and places are what often stand out in my memory, and alongside this the times when I have really had to put myself into situations that I have been terrified of. I worked in Germany with the nurses, midwives and health visitors in the armed forces over a period of two years; this was a time of great learning for me in so many ways. In fact all of my work abroad has been of some significant note. However, the important part of any national or international work is the consolidation that takes place once one has returned to home base. It is then that the real reflection and integration can take place. This is something that I am deeply involved in learning at the moment, and I realise that there are many lessons still waiting for me. My story is unfolding before me; sometimes I have a glimpse of what the next chapter will be, at other times I am aware of being a (not always willing) character in a larger plot.

Conclusion

What comes through all of these case studies is the determination of all five people to bring research into practice, to question the care that is being provided. Clearly this is not always easy, and sometimes paths have to be cut across territory between professions. All five have approached care with an openness to multi-disciplinary working and to the involvement of peer review from other disciplines. This non-parochial aspect of their work allows for a breadth of knowledge and influences to penetrate our traditions and indicates the necessary maturity for a true professional.

Key also to the success of our five researchers, and each case study reflects this, is the importance of good mentorship and professional support. As a profession we are now beginning to share more, to be more generous, than perhaps was always the case, and this is to be greatly welcomed. Finally, each person had a clear idea of what they needed in order to succeed, and stepped outside the norm to achieve it. A certain discipline also comes through the stories, such as making the necessary time to successfully complete studies and ensuring the right support mechanisms are there in supervisory roles.

If you feel a little despondent after reading these reflections – perhaps you have not got a higher degree and do not see, at this moment in time, the opportunity to register to work for one, or perhaps do not feel that you could achieve one, take heart. Do not for one moment consider that this bars you from getting involved in research. It doesn't. Research is a way of thinking. The child who constantly says 'why' is the early researcher. Sadly this questioning approach often gets suppressed by society in general and by over-taxed parents in particular. Health care providers, today more than ever before with high expectations and demands set against limited resources, need to question practices and to be certain that their contribution is sound. This does not require a degree or a diploma – but it does require interest and initiative. If this interest leads you to consider a more formal approach to research, career options today are vibrant with opportunities.

Capacity building in research and development is a priority in the NHS now, and as is demonstrated by Rafferty and Traynor (Chapter 2), initiatives are being put into place to facilitate this expansion. If you want to understand a little more, maybe just to put a toe in the water of research seas, make a connection with someone who knows a little more than you do. Take it step by step. See if there is any appeal for you beyond the professional requirement for questioning practices and being up to date. If there is, go for it! Find out what scholarships or grants are available to you, talk to your employer about joint appointments with the local university. Consider secondments which safeguard your income and clinical placement but allow time for greater depth of study. Write letters to awarding charities, most of which have websites. An excellent one which I am involved with, so I know first hand how it advises and facilitates newcomers to research, is the Florence Nightingale Foundation, which gives annual scholarships to fund research training, Often these first steps lead to employers' recognition of your particular interests and skills gained and new career options arise accordingly. As more practitioners involve themselves in research, such as by linking with the lead R&D person in their trust or by contacting the nearest university department of nursing studies and collaborating with them, so will the gap between academia and practice diminish and the one will serve the other more richly to the benefit of patients.

It would be easy for the reader to assume that the people featuring case studies above live rather sad lives, enmeshed in nursing and research, and breathing the rarefied gases of academe. This is not the case – they are all family-oriented people, they enjoy socialising and have a great deal of humour. I have the privilege of knowing them all, and know this to be true.

As for me – I have had a wonderful career in health research, and as I look back in semi-retirement, I see how blessed I was in mentorship and support. It was a source of some amazement when I left a minor public school with three O levels (English literature, English language and Art), this small success being attributable, I suspect, to my love of the poem 'The Lady of Shallott' which I knew by heart and which appeared as an exam question, neat handwriting and an interesting use of colour. Indeed the school had already suggested to my fee-paying parents that they were wasting their hard earned money! My parents were utterly un-academic and the idea that I would later achieve an MPhil and a PhD would have been laughed out of court. My early working life was as a salesgirl and it was a chance decision to go pony trekking in the Highlands that led to my finding myself working as an auxiliary nurse to pay for the trip. The culture shock from high fashion to bedpans was quite something, but for me it was a time of great significance and the seed was sown. A slice of determination mixed with passion, and so much is possible.

Key points

- A career in research is not out of the question – if it appeals, make enquiries.
- A career in research demands constant questioning and commitment.
- Good mentorship is crucial to stability and success.
- Be prepared to step outside of the norm.

References

Bryar, R.M. (2003) Practitioner research: An approach to developing research capacity in primary care. *NTResearch*, **8**(2): 101–15.

Carroll, L. (1982) *Alice in Wonderland.* London: Hodder and Stoughton.

Garrison, J. (1997) *Dewey and Eros. Wisdom and Desire in the Art of Teaching.* New York: Teachers College Press, Columbia University.

Kenkre, J.E. and Foxcroft, D.R. (2001) Career Pathways in Research. *Academic Nursing Standard*, **16**(7): 40–4.

Pooh bear (2002) *The Proverbial Pooh.* London: Egmont Books.

Shaw, G.B. (1903) Man and superman. *Maxims for Revolutionists: Reason.* Cambridge, MA: Cambridge University Press.

Whitman, W. (1871) Song of the Open Road. In McKay, D. *Leaves of Grass.* Philadelphia. Philadelphia PS 3201: Robarts Library.

8 Developing a research portfolio: Building a professional profile

Veronica Bishop and Dawn Freshwater

Neglect research and you neglect health. (WHO, 1992)

In this chapter the authors differentiate between the organisation portfolio and that of the individual. Set against current funding exercises and policy initiatives advice is given on how to contribute to the greater plan while accumulating personal growth. The need to keep research close to patient care is stressed and strategies for doing this are highlighted.

Introduction

There are two main strands to developing a research portfolio. The first to consider is that of the department or organisation where you work, the second is your personal portfolio which ideally (but not necessarily) is inextricably linked to the first. In this chapter we consider both the organisational and personal factors that contribute to the development of a themed research portfolio. We also stress the link between the building of an individual and organisational portfolio and the wider policy issues and national agendas. The chapter then considers how the individual researcher can engage in the dynamic interplay between continuing professional development, career pathways and organisational outcomes.

Organisational portfolios: The macro approach

Research activity within the nursing and midwifery professions can be identified in the UK since the early years of the National

Health Service. Concerns then focused mainly on the most appropriate use of staff resources – a debate which continues to today and undoubtedly will for decades to come as the NHS changes, technology advances and different skills are required to meet the health needs of the population. Early nursing research in the UK was funded by charitable organisations and attempted to undertake a fundamental analysis of the task of nursing (Menzies, 1959; Nuffield Provincial Hospitals Trust, 1953). In 1968 the Department of Health and Social Security was allocated funds to support research into nursing by commissioning a number of small-scale studies under common themes. For example, education, nursing and midwifery recruitment and retention issues, and career pathways were funded under the theme 'workforce'. These studies, usually sited within established university departments, then developed into longer-term programmes, using longitudinal studies often funded by what was termed a 'rolling contract'. Continuation of the contract was dependant on periodic satisfactory academic review. Directly commissioned shorter-term projects on nursing and midwifery issues have been ongoing in parallel with themed programmes. These studies are much more likely to provide local and contingent knowledge, offering valuable insights into specific contextual aspects of care.

The success of a programme of research will be measured, in the main, by the amount of funding it attracts (see Chapter 9 for a detailed description of research funding), by the number of peer reviewed publications that the staff involved have had published, and by the number of conferences presentations, particularly large national and international venues, where the study has been debated and developed. The number of students attracted to an institution, both pre- and post-graduate (depending on the educational remit of the organisation) will also have a bearing on the academic prestige allocated, particularly the successful completion of Masters and Doctoral awards. These indices are valued across the world and are, in the main, those used by the Research Assessment Rating Exercise in the UK. The score allocated to research departments reflects the percentage of further funding to be made available from the Higher Education Funding Council – until recently one of the main sources of monies for any university. This system has much to commend – it such as the attention to peer review and that it drives dissemination programmes and encourages the uptake of postgraduate students. However, there are as many critics of the system as there are proponents, not least owing to the fact that programmes are more likely to focus on short-term issues for quick results and little opportunity is easily available to seek knowledge for knowledge's sake, which may or may not have a foreseeable knock-on pragmatic outcome.

Funding bodies commissioning the research role will want to consider the quality and expertise of the institution or individual, ensuring that they have either a sound reputation in the subject to be investigated or a specific methodological area. This can make it difficult to break into a subject as a newcomer, despite sound academic qualifications and a solid team. There are a lot of hungry institutions chasing a very limited amount of funding, and the competition is fierce. Competition is useful in raising standards but is not always conducive to the development of a truly collegiate spirit. However, there are ways to overcome this, and currently many organisations commissioning studies encourage a multi-site collaborative approach. For example, national funds were recently made available for the development of a new role in primary mental health care, that of the graduate mental health worker. Regional collaboration was encouraged, with input from several higher education institutions, primary care trusts and workforce development confederations being favoured by the commissioners. Multi-site studies, which adhere strictly to the planned methodology, are common in medical research. The results of smaller studies (particularly quantitative studies) are often aggregated (combined) thus allowing statistical analysis and generalisability to a wider population. A study that took a similar approach was carried out to evaluate the effectiveness of the implementation of clinical supervision across 18 sites in England and Scotland (Butterworth et al., 1997), and while the study was flawed, owing to organisational limitations, the resultant interest and dissemination set the pace for a great deal of further locally driven work on clinical supervision (Freshwater et al., 2001, 2002); sadly, though, not as yet on another multi-site scale.

Given the brief background described above the challenges to developing a major research programme are self-evident in that funding sources are limited, programmes of research need to be policy or bio-medically oriented to attract funding from the major funding organisations, and acknowledged expertise in the selected field of study is expected. A further complexity in all social sciences research is that much of the nature of these disciplines is dependent on diffuse interactions and tacit understandings which do not lend themselves to clearly defined methodologies. In other words, the variables are not always controllable, thus making the gold standard of research methodology – quantitative experimentation – inappropriate. Added to these difficulties setting up a programme of research in nursing is perhaps more challenging than in many other health care subjects due to the enormity of the role of nursing. How does one decide, in a politically astute manner, the best way to investigate areas of education, clinical care and management and thus serve the two populations – the health care staff and the patients? The bottom line question is – what is nursing? Bishop (2001) holds the view that nursing is identified by the provision of professional, knowledgeable care. Whichever definition is preferred, it cannot be argued that while much of the work of nurses is very diffuse, the work, whatever the setting, draws upon a tradition of caring, based around both skills and values. In *Challenges for nursing and midwifery in the 21st century* (DoH, 1994) consideration is given to what these skills may be. They include:

- a co-ordinating function
- a teaching function for carers, patients and professionals
- developing and maintaining programmes of care
- technical expertise, exercised personally and through others
- concern for the ill, but also for those who are currently well
- a special responsibility for the frail and vulnerable.

In effect, an agenda is drawn up here which touches every aspect of health care, and it could be as appropriately pointed to medical colleagues as well as any of the professions allied to medicine. The issue is to select and develop complementary areas of expertise which can be sustained over a period of years. The importance of developing a programme of practice-based and cumulative research must be at the heart of a strategy for advancing research into nursing and allied professions. The government-driven agenda to health care may sometimes seem to exclude issues which pertain to nursing, and the dilemma of fitting nursing activities and interactions into rigid protocols has been much discussed (Lorentzen, 1995; Traynor and Rafferty, 1997) and has serious considerations for anyone involved in planning a research portfolio, as the Government is the largest R&D funding body. However, we are convinced that as long as the nursing aspects of any given programme are addressed there is the potential to build a portfolio which will not simply attract funding but importantly contribute to the body of nursing knowledge. For example, coronary heart disease is a current major issue which the Government is committed to, as it is to other serious and chronic diseases, as can be seen in the publication of the National Service Frameworks. Consider the 'nursing constants' listed above and it will be seen that there is not one function which could not be addressed within the context of coronary care. The same applies to cancer care services, paediatric, palliative care, mental health, and so on. There are many opportunities, though not without their own challenges. Developing a knowledge base which is applicable to any 'theme' in health care offers opportunities for all health care professionals, and importantly, highly valued niches for statisticians and health economists as well.

Academic research centres in practice

There are several models by which an organisation might go about building an institutional portfolio. One such example, of particular relevance to nursing practice, is that of the academic research centre in practice. A number of these are being developed across the south-east of England. Each centre is firstly tasked with identifying particular domains of knowledge and practice to create a focus for synthesising practice improvement, research and learning. This is being achieved through 'enabling work based learning, research and quality improvements to take place in relation to clinical practice and the priorities of the NHS' (Freshwater and Wallace, 2003:15). Whilst individual trusts benefit from the development of an academic centre in practice, as it assists in them in meeting a number of institutional objectives such as research governance, the university department also profits from such an initiative. Each centre establishes a focused research programme to evaluate both research, practice and educational activities, with a clear emphasis on improving the way services meet the needs of the trust's patients and the local community. Thus they are a very real example of partnership working at all levels and a useful model of how to develop both an institutional portfolio while focusing on what rally matters, the patient. The success of such an institutional centre can be distilled down to two influential factors, these being the need for strong and inspirational leadership, and the need for a focused programmatic approach to research. We come back to these two significant issues in our final discussion in Chapter 11.

Developing a personal research portfolio

A prospective pre-graduate student will consider the various universities that claim a particular expertise in the field that they wish to study, such as drama and the arts or sports, before selecting which one to attend. In the same way, a prospective researcher should consider what aspect of health care particularly interests him or her and consider carefully the options for further study. Different university departments develop their own areas of expertise, and it is much easier to study a subject where there is already a cadre of knowledgeable individuals who are likely to share and bolster your enthusiasm than to go it alone and against the flow of an established area of interest. However, it should also be noted that it is expected that at some point the researcher will develop new knowledge which challenges tried and trusted ways of understanding practice. One of the ways forward in the first instance is to become attached to an established team who address the subject you wish to study, and to gradually inject your own perspective and passion. If this does not seem possible then an alternative is to try to join a department with a good reputation and, supported by the collaborative academic credibility, dig your own path. Clearly support from peers is crucial, especially when the work being developed is at the edge of current thinking.

A common starting-point in a career in research is to become a research assistant in a department of nursing studies. Work at this level will build upon previous general education and on nursing skills in particular. Following or developing a specific interest in nursing and, where possible, increasing your input into that area of research is the beginning of a personal research portfolio. There will be opportunities to write reports which in turn will lead to collaborative single authorship of papers published. The art of developing a personal portfolio is to grasp every opportunity to stretch yourself, whether it is through data collection, data analyses, helping to develop protocols for funding bodies and ethics committees. As a general rule there is a generosity of spirit in academia which is demonstrated widely by the sharing of expertise freely, despite the competition for limited resources, which the new researcher will do well to emulate. Sharing such as through joint authorships, the sometimes tedious sorting of data, and so on will bring the best of academia close to your work and increase both your understanding and your contribution.

There are scholarships available, such as the Florence Nightingale annual awards to fund research education or the writing-up of theses phase, or to travel to see how care is organised abroad, and, as was mentioned in Chapter 3, there are also Harkness and Fulbright scholarships, to name a few. Such awards allow you to pursue your particular interest in a manner which is complementary to the aims of your employing organisation. The importance of international and national awards should not be underestimated – they indicate to the wider world that achievement of some significance has been marked, and such marks are beneficial to the development of any portfolio. The consideration of marked recognition raises the issue of curriculum vitae (CV). These records of professional and academic achievement are often thrown together with little thought of how helpful they are to the reader. Good spacing between activities and sections is helpful, and care as to the size and type of print used. Capitals are not conducive to continuous reading, neither is the use of italics or decorative writing. For a research-focused CV ensure that every presentation, international, and national, is recorded, that every publication, whether with joint authorship or single, is listed, and that any course successfully completed is noted. It is helpful if the most recent post held is listed first, after the front sheet with your name and personal details, and if the receding chronological order maintained throughout. This is a fine detail which word processors allow with little effort and which makes a great deal of difference to the interest of the reader. An eye to details like these will help to create a clear and appealing CV – a most important document, your stepping stone to new opportunities.

A degree of pragmatism is usually essential in forging a name for oneself in research. If you work in a department which is focused on manpower issues there may be little mileage in trying to carve a career for yourself in issues around, for example, patient nutrition – though no doubt there are those who could (and would) dispute this. The point that we wish to make, quite strongly, is that collaboration offers a far more research-conducive atmosphere than isolation. More to the point, if your work is not complementary to the main body of effort the rationale to keep you employed may go. Once you have established a name for yourself in a specific area, then the position may well change and you will be invited to dig your own furrow.

It is not always easy to follow one's chosen area, as can be read in Chapter 7. The case studies cited do not portray clear-cut routes, yet each subject, with a mixture of passion, determination and hard work, has carved out areas of expertise for him- or herself and brings to the professional body his or her unique contribution.

Supervision and support

We have previously highlighted the need for good supervision and support. Much of the success of any individual in achieving his or her professional and academic success will depend on careful thought as to what support mechanisms will maximise success. This cannot be overemphasised, a view shared by Lawton (1997) and Philips and Pugh (1987). Who is best placed to provide the necessary insights and expertise, comfort you when all seems too challenging, excite you when the work is becoming boring, as sometimes it does? Who can build the bridges between the different disciplines which you may be investigating, who is conversant with differing traditions with respect to the research processes? Whether you are the head of a school or department or a lone researcher within a trust or team, the need for a combination of mentorship, academic challenge and general belief in you and what you are trying to achieve is paramount. It may be too much to find all these talents in one person – look around, approach people. You will be amazed at the generosity of individuals; generally people are very flattered that they are perceived as having something extra to offer and are happy to rise to the invitation. For such relationships to be beneficial it is important that the inherent expectations are voiced rather than taken for granted. As Miller (1999:79) states, 'it is knowing what is required, when it is required and how to provide it that constitutes effective supervision'. Support and supervision in research are not about cosiness or constant positive strokes, conversely neither are they about being made to feel inadequate or stupid. There is a tremendous element of trust in any supervisory arrangement, whether it be in clinical supervision (Freshwater, 2001; Bishop, 1998) or academic activities. This trust is not only concerned with confidentiality but also with sensitivity to the supervisee's vulnerability when breaking new ground. It is tempting to select someone who will provide a bulletproof comfort zone to meet these last requirements but remember, your best friend is unlikely to be a suitable choice as a supervisor. However, it is quite possible that he or she becomes one at the end of a rigorous and successful journey together.

Academic support should be automatically built in to any collaborative arrangement with an institution of higher education. However, it must be admitted that these arrangements are more dependent on the individuals than the host academic department, and if insufficient access is offered then ask for a change of supervisor, even if it means upsetting the status quo. Not an easy thing to take on, but at the end of the day you are responsible for your work and it is you who will be judged by it, so be clear as to your needs.

Discussion

The need to keep much of nursing research close to the patient is imperative if nursing is to grow as a profession and bring intellectual activity to improve overall care provision. What has been described as the art and science of nursing (Marks Maran, 1999) needs to be explored and developed. It is with this aim in mind that the five individuals who are profiled in Chapter 7 broke new paths and made links with practice despite the pressures of academia. These days such opportunities are much easier to broker. The reasons for this are:

1. NHS care providers need to demonstrate that they are supporting staff in professional development and that they are good investors in people.
2. Employers need to be assured that their practices are sound.
3. Institutions of higher education need the financial gain accorded to them by collaboration with the NHS and the private sector.
4. None of them can function without the student – at whatever level. This gives the individual a great deal of power which, if used carefully, can broker enormously beneficial collaborative arrangements between the clinical settings and academia!

One word of caution, such arrangements may require a great deal of energy, with two 'masters' to be placated. Be sure that any arrangements are not setting you up to fail, with too little time for proper study, or inadequate clinical or academic support.

Key points

- Research requires personal commitment to professional knowledge.
- Be clear as to your role and your expectations in collaborative arrangements.
- Do not work in a strategic or personal vacuum.
- Joint partnerships can be beneficial at every level, from novice to professorial.

References

Bishop, V. (1998) *Clinical supervision, What is it? Some questions, answers and guidelines.* Basingstoke: MacMillan – now Palgrave Macmillan.

Bishop, V. (2001) *Challenges in clinical practice. Professional developments in nursing.* Basingstoke: Palgrave – now Palgrave Macmillan.

Butterworth, T., Carson, J., White, E., Jeacock, J., Clements, A. and Bishop, V. (1997) *It is good to talk. An evaluation study in England and Scotland.* Manchester: University of Manchester.

DoH (Department of Health) (1994) *Challenges for nursing and midwifery in the 21st century: the Heathrow debate.* London: HMSO.

Freshwater, D. (2001) Research and the reflective practitioner. In Rolfe, G., Freshwater, D. and Jasper, M. *Critical Reflection for Nursing and the Helping Professions. A Users' Guide.* London: Palgrave – now Palgrave Macmillan.

Freshwater, D. and Wallace, S. (2003) *Academic centres in practice.* The Beacon Bournemouth University Spring issue.

Freshwater, D., Walsh, L. and Storey, L. (2001) Developing leadership through clinical supervision in prison healthcare. *Nursing Management,* **8**(8): 10–13.

Freshwater, D., Walsh, L. and Storey, L. (2002) Developing leadership through clinical supervision in prison healthcare. *Nursing Management,* Feb.

Lawton, D. (1997) How to succeed in postgraduate study. In Graves, N. and Varia, V. (eds) *Working for a doctorate.* London: Routledge.

Lorentzen, M. (1995) Guest editorial, multidisciplinary collaboration. Life-line or drowning pool for nurse researchers? *Journal of Advanced Nursing,* **22**(5): 825.

Marks-Maran D., (1999) Reconstructing nursing: evidence, artistry and the curriculum. *Nurse Education Today,* **19**, 3–11.

Menzies, I.E.P. (1959) The functioning of social systems as a defence against anxiety. A report of a study of the nursing services of a general hospital. *Human Relations,* **13**: 95–121.

Miller, R. (1999) Supervisor's comments. In Bishop, V. (ed.) *Working towards a research degree. Insights into the nursing perspective.* London: Emap publications.

Nuffield Provincial Hospitals Trust (1953) *The work of nurses in hospital wards.* London: Nuffield Provincial Hospitals Trust.

Philips, E.M. and Pugh, D.S. (1987) *How to get a PhD.* Milton Keynes: Open University Press.

Traynor, M. and Rafferty, A.M. (1997) *The NHS R&D context for nursing research: a working paper.* London: School of Hygiene and Tropical Medicine, Centre for Policy in Nursing Research.

WHO (World Health Organisation) (1992) *Research Strategies for Health.* Geneva: WHO.

9 Funding for Nursing Research: Writing grant applications

Dawn Freshwater

Whether you are embarking upon a research degree, a looking for an opportunity to develop your clinical practice or working as part of a team in academe, the issue of funding is likely to be something that demands your attention. Whilst funding options and interests vary according to your starting position there are some fundamental principles which should be understood and addressed. This chapter focuses on the skills of writing for funding but, importantly, outlines the context within which nursing seeks such funding. Current policies in nursing and research are examined in the light of academic developments.

Introduction

Most substantial research projects require some financial support. This might be for personnel (for example the appointment of a research assistant or buying out existing staff from their current role), equipment or publication/dissemination costs. Few departments can support the development of research from within their existing budgets, which are already stretched to the limit. In addition, research is often seen as low on the list of priorities when it comes to investing money. Thus an important part of research activity is learning to write research proposals for research funding, with the skill of writing a grant application being as important as the skills of enquiry themselves. The skills of proposal writing are just as important in the context of studying for a higher degree. In the context of higher-level study, an approved proposal constitutes a bond of agreement between the student and the supervisor and the department or academic school. In the research funding context an approved grant application results in a contract between the investigator and a funding source.

Funding bodies

Page (1999:25) describes the changing political and professional landscape and the concomitant increased appreciation (desperation) of the need to 'grow' more nurses educated to doctoral level. She highlights several options in searching for funding sources, particularly for the would-be PhD student. Options range from the employer, though this is rare, DoH R&D funding, charities, the research councils and statutory bodies. There are a number of institutions that provide funding specifically for nurses, including the Smith and Nephew Foundation, the Florence Nightingale Foundation, the Foundation of Nursing Studies and the Queens Nursing Institute. Whatever your status, be it a would-be post graduate student or a qualified researcher, the value of taking your time to establish funding links, to identify relevant issues and to feel within the enthusiasm for the subject to successfully conclude the proposed work cannot be underestimated.

Funding for research in nursing

Over the last two decades there have been a number of papers that have set out the performance of nursing research (see, for example, Kitson, 1997; Greenwood, 1984; Mead, 1996; Rafferty, Bond and Traynor, 2000). Writers have, by and large, reached the same conclusion, that 'the amount and quality of research in nursing is improving, but the base remains low' (Mead and Mosely, 2000:39). There was hope that, with the move of nursing in higher education (HE), nursing research would at last come into its own. However, neither the NHS nor the HE sector assumed the responsibility for the funding of nursing research. Traditionally funding for research in HE has come from two main sources, the funding councils and the research councils. Mead and Mosely (2000:40) explain that

> The intention is that these two sources provide institutions with funding for their basic infrastructure, which supports a research capacity. The funding councils fund staff, equipment, and facilities, such as laboratories and libraries, accommodation and so on, in other words the basic infrastructure for carrying out research. The research councils provide funding for work on specific projects at specific times, for example research staff and specialised equipment for a given project.

There has however been no nursing research council, although nurses have been encouraged to apply to the Medical Research Council (MRC) and the Economic and Social Research Council (ESRC) for finance, with, it has to be said, limited success. Further, nursing has had little call on the funding councils, having underachieved in the Research Assessment Exercise (RAE).

As has been discussed at earlier points in this book, the NHS Research and Development strategy that was developed over ten years ago demonstrated the Government's commitment to fund and support research that was of direct relevance to the service. As Traynor, Rafferty and Spragg (2002) point out, the Government was also keen to ensure that research funds were used appropriately by researchers rather than their being driven by the researchers' own interests and priorities. Since then the drive for nurses and allied health professions to better understand and appraise research findings in the pursuit of evidence-based practice has led to significant changes. Concurrently there has been a growing body of evidence to support the anecdotal reports that the nursing research infrastructure was enormously underdeveloped (Centre for Policy in Nursing Research, 2001).

In 1994 a report published by the Department of Health laid out recommendations for a reorganisation of the relationships between the NHS, higher education institutions and special funding councils in order that research directly relevant to the NHS could be fostered. As Curzio (1998) notes, this aim of this report was also to ensure the research component of the NHS budget be better identified 'and managed for the benefit of the health service' (p. 103). Following this report organisations were encouraged to tender for ring-fenced monies to support the development of a research portfolio or programme.

More recently Traynor et al. (2002) and Rafferty et al. (2000, see also Chapter 2) report pleasing developments in the funding of nursing research. Two major funding organisations of research have been focusing on the deficit in the research capacity of both nursing and allied health professions. Both the Department of Health and the PPP foundation (formerly the PPP Healthcare Medical Trust) have made substantial financial commitments to the development of new research initiatives. Additionally the NHS Service and Delivery Organisation (SDO) has ring-fenced funds for research conducted by nurses into the NHS service delivery. More recently HEFCE have added to this, with the money being used specifically to support the development of the research capacity in nursing. HEFCE has also announced two new award schemes to develop future nursing research leaders. These are the researcher development award (for nurses of outstanding potential early on in their research career) and the postdoctoral award (for nurses who lack the required experience in independent research) (see Chapter 1; Scott, 2002). The challenge now is for nurse researchers to turn nursing into a discipline of international repute. This requires a dramatic thrust in the support and development of the capacity of nurse researchers to bid competitively for research funds. And, of course, there are substantial implications for the generation of educational packages to enable the nursing professions as a whole to acquire the skills to meet this challenge. Writing grant applications is one such skill.

Writing for research funding

The English National Board, in 1998, contended that conducting nationally funded research was one of the most important ways of contributing to the delivery of effective health care. Guidelines were produced by the ENB intended to help researchers identify the key issues and pitfalls in pulling together a research proposal. They emphasised three overall aims to be taken into consideration when working on a grant application, these being the clarity of the research process, the generalisability or transferability of the findings of the study and the familiarity and expertise of the research team with the subject (ENB, 1995). The following section outlines in more detail the process of writing a grant application.

Applications for funding, known as grant applications, are formal appeals for an award of support through a contract with a grantor who has a special interest (Locke, Psirduso and Silverman, 1993). Grants may be sought to undertake a specific project in which the objective is to provide and perhaps evaluate a service and its added value. Grants are also available that aim to generate knowledge that might influence the later development of a service. A grant application normally consists of two main components, the first being the application for funding, the second an in-depth proposal that details the activities to be supported. In this way a grant application necessitates the same skills as the preparation of a research proposal. However, when writing a grant proposal the researcher is required to conform to the specific requests of the commissioning body as well as to demonstrate that the research team has the skills to deliver the project to a high standard. As we have already discussed (see Chapter 6) the best evidence of competence is dissemination through conference papers and publications in peer-reviewed journals – that is, evidence of a research track record. A strong track record in research is important, in that many fundholders make decisions about allocation of funds based on the history of the applicants, although there are also a number of institutions that use a blind review process. However, as mentioned above, when reviewing grant applications review panels take into account other factors in addition to track record, for example the significance of the research question and its fit with the grantors' agenda. Further, each funding body has a unique form to be completed and processes differ across and within organisations. Understanding of these processes, and of the agenda of the organisation, can be helpful to the novice researcher.

Writing proposals for funding then can be a very time consuming and not always rewarding experience. The ratio of proposals funded to those being rejected is very low. In 1993 Locke et al. suggested that 'fewer than 30% of first time applicants to the National Institutes of Health are successful' (p. 147). The reality is that this is not likely to be very much different ten years later, in fact with more researchers chasing fewer funds it is probably even tighter. However, this is not to say that grant applications are not worth pursuing, but it is important to be realistic in your aspirations and to familiarise yourself with smaller local sources that are often easier to access as well as some of the larger national funds that are much sought after. Obtaining small locally funded grants can provide useful start-up costs for a research project that is more likely to gain further funding once the main ideas have been tested. As Locke et al. (1993) point out: 'In programmatic research it is logical sequence not the accumulated number of studies, that will impress reviewers' (p. 148).

A successful research proposal will excel in its ability to communicate the investigators intentions and research plans.

Maxwell (1996) and Punch (2000) argue that the form and structure of the proposal are tied to its purpose, this being 'to explain and justify your proposed study to an audience of non-experts on your topic' (Maxwell, 1996:100–1). Punch (2000) states that the proposal also acts as an action plan for carrying out the research. There are numerous descriptions of how to write research proposals, and examples of grantmanship.

Questions to consider when formulating the proposal are:

- Who will read the proposal?
- What are their expectations?
- What is the process for approval of the proposal?
- What departmental guidelines should be adhered too?

Suggested proposal headings (in numbered order) are:

1. Title and title page
2. Abstract
3. Introduction
4. Research questions
5. Conceptual framework
6. The literature
7. Methodology
8. Significance
9. Consent and ethical concerns
10. References
11. Appendices.

Each of these will be briefly addressed in turn.

Title and abstract

Titles are often dictated when applying for formally commissioned research funds, however when a general call is answered the title is obviously of significance, being the first thing that the review panel will see. Locke et al. (1993:162) note that the document that does not 'catch the eye – and thus the reward of closer attention and consideration – cannot compete on the formal criteria associated with quality of design and congruence with the grantor's priorities'. For this reason the quality of both the abstract and the introduction is paramount. The abstract provides the reviewer with a brief summary of the proposed study. Abstract writing is a skill in itself, requiring the skill of saying a lot in a few words. Each word and sentence must communicate a precise message to the reviewer. For a grant application the abstract needs to explicate what the study is about, what it aims to achieve and how it intends to do it.

Introduction

The introduction sets the stage for the research and is the lead-in for the reader. As Punch (2000:69) points out: 'Its purpose is not to review the literature, but rather to show generally how the proposed study fits into what is already known, and to locate it in relation to present knowledge and practice.' There are four key components to an introduction:

1. establishing the problem leading to the development of the study
2. locating the problem within the larger scholarly literature
3. identifying gaps in the literature about the problem
4. targeting an audience and observing the significance of this problem for the audience.

(adapted from Cheswell, 1994).

Research questions

Often the research questions are predetermined; however, the nature and the central role of the research question needs to be discussed. Where the research question is one that has been determined by the research team, a full and detailed background to the emergence of the question should be provided (refer to earlier chapters in this book).

Conceptual framework and literature

The proposal needs to identify both the conceptual framework and the body of literature which is relevant to the research question. Thus indicating the relationship of the study to the broader literature (see Chapter 3).

Methodology

The research methodology connects the research question to the data, detailing the implementation of the research strategy. There are a number of methodological and theoretical factors to consider when writing the application.

- The research team needs to demonstrate the relevance of the research topic in the wider context of nursing and health care.
- The overall intention of the research needs to be clear.
- Explicit reference should be made to the extent to which the proposed research will contribute to the understanding of the problem.
- The methodological framework provides a link between the overall design of the project, the data collection, the data analysis and the presentation of the findings.
- The research team should indicate the sampling strategy, the extent of the proposed sample and how the sample units will be chosen.
- A brief description of the data collection and data analysis techniques should be provided.

Significance

This is the point at which the researcher indicates the importance or contribution of the study, answering the basic question: Why is the study worth doing? In answering this question it is not just the contribution of new knowledge (often interpreted as the theoretical contribution) that drives research, and as such it is prudent to refer to the relative merits for policy makers and, importantly, practitioners. Funding agencies are accountable to the public and to their benefactors for the appropriate expenditure of their funds and, while this aspect of the proposal might not be lengthy, it deserves focused attention.

Consent and ethical concerns

All individuals involved in research are expected to be cognisant of the four ethical principles: the respect for autonomy; the principle of non-maleficience; the principle of beneficence; and the principle of justice. Grant applications and research proposals in general are expected to make explicit the arrangements for gaining informed consent from participants and ways in which the researcher will minimise any potential harm to those involved. Other ethical rules should also be attended to within the process such as privacy, confidentiality, truth telling and faithfulness.

References and Appendices

In addition to a list of references, the appendices will include a timetable for the research, the proposed budget, consent and ethical approval forms. Examples of questionnaires, interview guides and findings from pilot studies may also be included. The appendices then can demonstrate that the researcher has given due consideration to other important practical considerations including providing evidence of practical project management demonstrated through a realistic time-scale and a full account of financial planning, including staff and non-staff costs (such as travel expenses, institutional overheads and postage).

It is virtually guaranteed that one of your proposals, at some point, will be rejected. Locke et al. (1993) observe that reasons for rejection of proposals generally fall into one or more of four categories: mechanical, methodological, personnel and cost benefit. Although, of course, it is also the case that perfectly sound proposals can also be rejected, there are often some basic errors that can be avoided with deliberate and focused attention on the task in hand.

The following are common reasons for rejection of research proposals (adapted from Locke et al., 1993):

1. *Mechanical*
   - Guidelines for submission were not followed.
   - The proposal did not clearly outline one or several elements of the study.
   - The quality of writing was poor.
   - The document contained an excessive number of mechanical defects reflecting the carelessness of the researcher.

2. *Methodological*
   - The proposed method of study was unsuited to the purpose of the research.
   - The method offered nothing new, intriguing or striking in relation to the research topic.

3. *Personnel*
   - The researcher did not understand or have sufficient knowledge of the territory.
   - The proposal seems to be beyond the capacity of the research team.

4. *Cost–benefit reasons*
   - The proposed budget was unrealistic either in terms of estimated requirements or its possible benefit to the service.

Rejection is not a good feeling for anyone, however once the initial disappointment is over, the researcher should not be put off from searching for other funding for the same project, nor from writing subsequent research grants.

Dissemination of results

Professional and practical issues in regard to dissemination have been addressed in earlier chapters and indeed throughout the book. Of course, the book itself is an example of dissemination and, while it is not possible for everyone to be engaged in substantial writing projects, it is important that practitioners take responsibility for improving not only their own practice but also potentially that of others.

Responsibility

Taylor (2003) notes the politics of social research and identifies that responsibility emerges as a core category in funded research. She argues that researchers are responsible to and for the following:

- the organisation that has commissioned the research
- other stakeholders who are involved with the funding
- the researchers themselves
- their profession
- the beneficiaries of the research for example the community and patients
- the academic community.

As Taylor points out, pleasing everyone and having many masters becomes complex, and is often challenging. Clarity of the inherent tensions that any proposed work may invoke and staying close to the integrity of the methodology and the resultant analysis are important factors, as is of course keeping key stakeholders informed through steering groups and regular reports. As Bishop (2003) notes often those commissioning research do not have the relevant expertise to realise either the limitations of a proposed study nor the capacity to accept findings which may be unpopular.

Conclusion

Whilst the news regarding the funding of nursing research is currently very positive, with more and more professional staff keen to carry out funded research and a growing number of experience nurse researchers, the competition will continue to be fierce. It is therefore important to maximise the likelihood of obtaining research funding. In order to do so Curzio (1998) suggests, and this text has reiterated, the following:

- collaborating with other experienced researchers who have a track record of obtaining funding
- developing the skills of writing robust research proposals that can withstand critical appraisal
- developing a personal/professional portfolio of sustained research activity.

Key points

- Resources for nursing research are scarce and the competition great.
- Clarity of research proposals is essential.
- Understanding of stakeholders' perspectives is necessary.
- Collaboration can be beneficial, particularly for the novice.

References

Bishop, V. (2003) Review: *NTResearch*, in press.

Centre for Policy in Nursing Research, R&D Forum Allied Health Professions, Association of Commonwealth Universities, CHEMS Consulting (2001) *Promoting Research in Nursing, Midwifery, Health Visiting and Allied Health Professions: Report to DH/HEFCE Taskgroup 3*. Bristol: Higher Education Funding Council for England.

Cheswell, J.W. (1994) *Research Design: Qualitative and Quantitative Approaches*. Thousand Islands: California.

Curzio, J. (1998) Funding for Evidence Based Practice in the UK. *NTResearch*, **3**(2): 100–7.

ENB (English National Board for Nursing, Midwifery and Health Visiting) (1995) *National consultation to identify research priorities in Nursing, Midwifery and Health Visiting education and practice*. Report of the consultation and outcomes, London: ENB.

ENB (English National Board for Nursing, Midwifery and Health Visiting) (1998) *Getting research funded, guidelines for preparing research proposals*. London: English National Board for Nursing, Midwifery and Health Visiting.

Greenwood, J. (1984) Nursing research: A position paper. *Journal of Advanced Nursing*, **9**: 77–82.

Kitson, A. (1997) Lessons from the 1996 Research Assessment Exercise. *Nurse Researcher*, **4**(3): 81–93.

Locke, L.F., Psirduso, W.W. and Silverman, S.J. (1993) *Proposals that work*. 3rd edn, California: Sage.

Maxwell, J.A. (1996) *Qualitative research design: An interactive approach*. Thousand Oaks: California.

Mead, D.M. (1996) Using nursing initiatives to encourage the use of nursing research. *Nursing Standard*, **10**(19): 33–6.

Mead, D. and Moseley, L. (2000) Developing nursing research in a contract driven arena: inequities and iniquities. *Nursing Standard*, October 25, **15**(6): 39–43

Page S. (1999) Funding for nurses. In. Bishop, V. (ed.) *Working Towards a Research Degree*. London: Emap Publications.

Punch, K.F. (2000) *Developing Effective Research Proposals*. London: Sage.

Rafferty, A.M., Bond, S. and Traynor, M. (2000) *Measuring the outputs of nursing R&D: A third working paper*. London: Centre for Policy in Nursing Research and London School of Hygiene and Tropical Medicine.

Scott, G. (2002) Funding boost is on the way for nursing research. *Nursing Standard*, May 22, **16**(36): 6.

Taylor, J. (2003) Politics or Paranoia; Reading between the lines when undertaking social research studies. *NT Research*.

Traynor, M., Rafferty, A.M. and Spragg, J. (2002) Cash Backing. *Nursing Standard*, December 18, **17**(14–15): 72.

10 Knocking down ivory towers: Publish and be dammed

Veronica Bishop

A little knowledge that acts is worth infinitely more than much knowledge that is idle. (Khalil Gibran, 1965)

In this chapter the importance of getting work published and moving research from paper to practice is stressed. Advice is offered for both the beginner and the more experienced on how to achieve this and the need to relate meaningfully with the rest of the health care professions is stressed.

Introduction

Dissemination is the vital link between research, development and changing practices. New knowledge generated from research and which has the potential to improve care delivery needs to be made accessible to the practitioners who can utilise it and to the managers who can facilitate change in practice and policy (Scottish Executive, 2002). This chapter highlights the importance of building bridges across the perceived practice and research gap and consideration is given to the reasons why clinical nurses may be reluctant to embrace research as part of their everyday practice. The emotional labour of clinical work is discussed, particularly in the context of organisational changes, evidence-driven care and the role of the practitioner–researcher in overcoming negative attitudes to research. The importance of practitioners making their own private knowledge public through dissemination of all sorts, particularly through publication, is stressed, with advice given on how to get material published, taking into account the types of publications for different audiences.

Ethical and social dimensions of making a difference

The importance of enquiry in nursing was first documented by Florence Nightingale in the 1860s (Nightingale, 1980) but as a profession nursing has been slow to grasp this concept as Simpson (1971) and later Salvage (1998) noted. Perhaps the hierarchical approach adopted from Nightingale is counterproductive to a problem-solving approach to care. The Foundation of Nursing Studies, an organisation dedicated to supporting nurses in bringing evidence-based care to patients and clients, carried out a study of workshops which they had organised to discuss the implementation of research findings into practice (FoNs, 1996). Many of the delegates questioned on their own practices held very estranging views of research. These perceptions included a 'them and us' approach, which viewed researchers as distant from day-to-day work, and some saw research activity as merely 'trendy' or irrelevant. While the reasons for this dismal approach to research is well documented elsewhere in this book, it is important to this chapter to consider the role of the report writer and disseminator in overcoming these attitudes.

There are those researchers who are deeply suspicious of efforts to increase the use of research, arguing that an increasingly utilitarian approach to research is likely to prove detrimental to the growth of knowledge in a wider sense (Richardson, Jackson and Sykes, 1990). This utilitarian approach can certainly limit the attention and funding allocated to research into narrow issues which meet short-term strategies. However, the fact remains that if research studies are not disseminated in a user-friendly way the work, however ground breaking, will not be implemented, the resources which have been used will be wasted, and the researcher's personal development will be limited. Most importantly of all, the opportunity to make a difference will be lost.

The phrase 'making a difference' has been used a great deal in nursing over the past eight years, and was initiated by the DoH document *Making a Difference* (DoH, 1999). Undertaking research at any level is about making a difference, whether it be at a local level or in the hope of making a much wider impact, for example by changing the way an area of health care is provided.

Making that extra effort of seeing a research project through from concept to analysis has a profound effect on any individual, and that person will thereafter bring to any situation a wider and more considered approach. The educational processes are never lost, though the detail may be soon forgotten. So, on a personal level, the difference may be intrinsic, bedded into the psyche, and the use of research may be so subtle that no direct connection to a particular project can be traced, but nevertheless professional practice is transformed. None the less we can never be complacent as there is no point of arrival in research; by its very nature it is a constant journey of lifelong learning. But it is a journey full of colour, offering great rewards which will be evidenced in many different ways, such as through increased confidence, a more reflective approach to problem solving, greater assertiveness, less aggression, and so on. However, making a difference within the wider health care arena will require further effort. Research cannot be used unless it is available to those who might use it, and for some this presents the greatest challenge – writing the report.

There are ethical, legal and practical issues around report writing, and all need a great deal of consideration. Ethics consent must be given from the appropriate formal ethics committee prior to any study being undertaken which involves staff, patients or their carers, and families. This is essential whether the study involves invasive procedures such as the taking of bloods, or non-invasive procedures such as making observational notes and the use of questionnaires. A further ethical dimension to undertaking research is that of sharing the research findings. There is a view that the researcher is beholden to make available data obtained from public goodwill and co-operation, whether or not the information will be pleasing. This can present difficulties to the researcher who may have been funded to undertake a study by policy makers who then are unhappy with the findings, a situation in which I have found myself involved in the past. On that occasion researchers had been funded by the Department of Health to undertake a skill mix study. Findings indicated that optimum care was provided when qualified nurses were involved in the care planning and processes, a view not favoured with the government of the time (Carr-Hill et al., 1992). As the commissioning officer for the DoH I went to extensive lengths to ensure the rigour of the work before it was made public. Scientific rigour is the principle which must apply to all research, be it quantitative or qualitative. However, it is recognised that different methodological approaches have different criteria to ensure rigour, an important issue more fully addressed in Chapter 4. Once validity is assured there is then a duty to share, to disseminate, to inform and teach. There is an expectation, particularly in qualitative work which uses co-operative enquiry in which the participants are seen as equal contributors and generators of the findings, that the overall effort will be rewarded by recognition through dissemination and by implementation of change for the better. Regrettably, this is not always the case.

Partnerships with practice

'Research can make a contribution to nursing services, practice, and education problems. It is important that such research should be continuously in progress and that well-established channels of communication exist to ensure that the end products of research are made swiftly available to the people who provided the service' (Simpson, 1971). Marjorie Simpson was an early doyen of research into nursing in the UK and yet, over thirty years later, the nursing profession as a whole still regards research as somewhat external to everyday practice. So why doesn't research get used very much in nursing? A symposium on clinical effectiveness (*NTResearch*, 1998) highlighted that many nurses lack confidence in research and in interpreting the results of research. This is something that educationalists need to be mindful of in planning future nursing curricula. It was agreed that development feeds research and that the converse is also true; however, to bridge this gap between practice and research it is necessary that research and implementation of its findings should be a part of everyone's job. This does not mean that everyone should undertake research, but that every practitioner should have access to research findings and be able to critique research reports. A progress report a of strategy to develop a partnership between a university and an acute trust (Martin et al., 1998) highlighted the importance of nursing research leaders and their role in sustaining, locally, the level of enthusiasm and commitment already evident. How can this be maintained? The relationship between service providers and researchers offers enormous potential for rich and exciting partnerships, and while creating a research culture throughout the health care services will not happen overnight, strategies employed to this end are to be applauded and supported.

The researcher–practitioner model (Freshwater and Rolfe, 2001) sees everyone as being involved in research and development with a small 'r' if they are approaching practice using critical reflexivity. However, as the Foundation of Nursing study mentioned above indicates, the relationship between researchers and practice development is often not a close one. In fact the difficulties in getting people to change their practice are legion. Nurses who do question practice are sometimes told dismissively that 'it's how we do things here'. It is difficult to persuade anyone to change from tried and known methods of care to new ways, particularly if the literature around the subject is woolly, unclear or full of jargon! The keen practitioner who comes in fresh with enthusiasm for recent research which challenges previous practices is liable to be looked at with scorn – with a 'who does she/he think they are' attitude – witness the continued difficulty in implementing clinical supervision and critical reflection. Challenging the norms is not easy in an already established culture.

Perhaps if the phrase 'emotional labour of nursing' were better understood the would-be researcher/writer would approach the task quite differently when attempting to address clinical colleagues. Certainly the work of Smith (1992) indicates that emotional labour provides a language with which to describe and investigate what are often seen as tacit and uncodified skills associated with care. The phrase is described by James (1993:95) as intended to highlight the similarities as well as differences between emotional and physical labour, with both being hard, skilled work requiring experience, affected by immediate conditions and external controls, and subject to divisions of labour. It is an integral yet often unrecognised part of employment that involves contact with people. This goes back to the work of Menzies (1970:1988) and Hochschild (1983) who suggest that emotional labour involves the induction or suppression of feeling in order to sustain an outward appearance that produces in others a sense of being cared for in a convivial safe place. Freshwater (1998, 2002) takes this concept further in the therapeutic use of self in nursing, saying that ' through the unfolding experience of reflection the nurse is looking backwards to the future, she is becoming while being (Freshwater 1998:16). This professional development may at times demand a façade, developed mainly for the benefit of others, and must carry a cost. I would suggest that one of its effects may result in a protection of armour plating against change, not least when so many organisational changes are inflicted in clinical areas over which the staff have no control. Given this less than comfortable scenario health care staff must be approached in a manner which offers a sympathetic connection to the world of enquiry. No one wants to feel that they are out of date, no one wants to be seen as second best – an outsider in a brave new world of research which perhaps they do not perceive that they have access to. Whilst a great deal of work has been carried out on why research findings are poorly implemented in nursing, and the reasons are well rehearsed not least within this book (with much of the fault lying at the feet of the organisation and culture within institutions), this aspect of feeling 'outside' is neglected. As for the organisational responsibilities, if obtaining research findings in your area of care is not explicitly stated as a part and parcel of your job, if the time and library facilities are not close by, then you may 'forget' that you have a statutory duty to be up to date, to question your practice and to promote best care, or, to put it more kindly, you may choose to presume that best practice prevails. Further, if a clinical environment is not supportive in terms of embracing changes in practice the practitioners may lack confidence in doing so, as was found in a study on an intervention to manage breathlessness (Froggatt, Corner and Bredin, 2002). This study identified that, while researchers focused on the production of new knowledge to create the evidence base upon which practice is taken forward, there were issues of the confidence of practitioners to take on new approaches. So what can you in your role as a researcher do to change this? How can you overcome the attitudinal and organisational barriers which prevent research from being utilised?

Publishing and dissemination

Hicks (1995; 1994) states that there is a shortfall of published nursing research and considers it to be due to a lack of confidence rather than a failure of nurses to conduct research. Despite this shortfall nursing research is one of the fastest-growing fields of biomedical and health research, indeed this is reflected in the expanding number of nursing journals (Rafferty, Traynor and Lewison, 2000). Health care research cannot be undertaken merely to promote the individual researcher – it must relate to service delivery in some way (see Chapter 8 on developing a research profile). However, such a diverse marketplace can confuse the novice would-be author, and time spent carefully considering who makes up the audience to be addressed and through which journal are they best found is time well spent. The words 'research report' do not resonate with excitement, do they? Not for the writer, as a rule, and certainly not for the reader. And indeed writing a report can be a stage in the research process that is the most difficult. How to infuse the written words with the excitement and relevance of your work without burying its essence in turgid detail when trying to indicate the scientific rigour applied to the study? This is not generally a talent granted at birth, but one worked at assiduously. However, it is effort which can be well rewarded (though rarely through financial gain) and is crucial for successful utilisation of the findings. A report or research paper can engender tremendous excitement if written with care and with the different prospective readers in mind. Tarling (1998) considers that there are, apart from the need to share good practices, several political reasons why you should seriously consider publishing the results of any study carried out. Resources, she points out, are limited and the researcher's life can be quite difficult at the best of times, publication is good for the curriculum vitae and, as stated earlier, the process of peer review is invaluable, adding another dimension to your work. This puts a great deal of responsibility on the author of the report who, in the early stages of his or her career, is unlikely to have had much practice in this area. Bogdan and Biklen (1982:172) describe the problems well when they state that 'novice writers are big procrastinators. They find countless reasons not to get started. Even when they finally get themselves seated at their desks, they always seem to find diversions: make the coffee, sharpen the pencil, and go to the bathroom'. Remember that you will not always be 'ready' to write; writing is something you must make a conscious decision to do and then discipline yourself to follow through.

The inclusion of an executive summary is helpful to the majority of readers and of course can be produced separately as well. Very few executives read more than the aims, abstract and conclusions, so a summary which very briefly takes them through the research process and highlights the essentials is much appreciated. Don't go overboard on the recommendations; a long list just irritates possible champions whereas a succinct list of less than ten is much more likely to get attention.

Approaches to be used in report writing vary to suit the potential reader. For example, a report on a study commissioned and funded by an external party, such as the Department of Health, would need to adopt a formal style in order to accommodate both the external scientific reviewers and the language of the Civil Service. While current trends in government communications are far less contrived than just half a decade ago, the scientific reviewers will need assurance that the work is properly and fully documented. Here the provision of an executive summary is invaluable and generally expected now. However, if the findings of a study are to be shared with a larger population, such as clinical nurses working in a particular speciality, then it is important to consider which magazines/journals they are most likely to read and to seek publication there. Publishing houses have different styles of layout and referencing, and to help would-be authors they usually produce guidelines for authors, either in each issue or on request. The two major referencing systems used in the UK are the Vancouver system, which places a number beside a reference within the text, and then lists references in numeric order at the end of the paper, and the Harvard system which brackets the name and date within the text and lists the references alphabetically at the end of the paper.

All references should be properly sourced, and if more than one is used to illustrate a point then they should be listed in the text in date order – usually the most recent being the first. Do not be fooled into thinking that referencing is unimportant because the reference list comes at the end of a paper or article – it is crucial to properly conducted work and important in acknowledging the work of others. A good example of referencing is given at the back of every issue of *Nursing Times Research* in its guide to authors (Emap Publications). Having written the research report in a manner which is appropriate for the funding body, educational institution or host establishment, consideration needs to be applied to the most appropriate way to disseminate your work further. Consent may be needed for this if the work was funded, for while the intellectual property of material on which you have worked is yours, the data may belong to the paymaster – a tricky relationship and one that needs careful negotiation.

Assuming that there are no restrictions and that you are free to publish and be read by a wider audience, how to choose which journal? First consider why you are publishing, then where. For example, the weekly professional magazines currently available to nurses have house styles which lend themselves to a 'quick read', unlike the more academically prestigious research and development journals which in general demand a more attentive perusal. The former will be ideal to bring issues to the attention of many, without too much detail, the latter will more advantageous in attracting a good rating in the overall academic review system, and possibly help the author to become established as an expert in his or her chosen field. As a general rule it is better to publish one solid paper of around 5000 words rather than two or three short articles. However, having published the substantive paper it is a very good move in terms of dissemination subsequently to extract several short papers referring back to the original work. Modes of dissemination include:

- final project report
- referenced papers in peer review journals
- seminars and conferences
- publication in books (as a chapter)
- short articles in speciality journals
- in-house journals
- websites

Clarity and style

Whichever publishing source you decide to seek, it is important to be clear as to what the message is in the work that you are going to present. Some writers advise writing the last paragraph first so that you are quite clear as to the course the paper is to take. Certainly deciding on which conclusions you are going to share dictates the course of the argument to be presented. Your chance to express yourself should not be wasted, so don't lose your reader with jargonistic style or repetitive sentences. Keep the essence of your message (what I call the primary colour or key thread) running throughout. Remember, the reader is unlikely to know why you decided to study the subject you are describing. The why, the how and the results are your primary colour, the rest is complementary shading. It may be helpful to make a list of topics which must be included in the overall text – key words – and while your family may not appreciate it, read the text out loud. It is amazing how, particularly with word-processing, one can type sentences leaving out essential verbs. Finally put the writing away in a drawer and leave it alone for week or so, if time allows. The improved objectivity that this brings is well worth the delay. Another very helpful tip is to find a colleague or academic whom you can approach and who is used to writing, and to ask for their critical review. When you are immersed in a subject, full of enthusiasm and, frankly, tunnel-visioned, a fresh perspective is essential. Share your enthusiasm with someone who has what you may lack – experience in crafting words. They will no doubt be heartened by your fresh energy and flattered by your approach to them for assistance. Don't be put off by what may appear to be a trashing of your effort.

It is the eagerness of the novice writer that persuades Albert (2000) that more people should have a go at publishing. He states that while knowledge and scholarship are important they need to be supplemented with enthusiasm, a quality that often seems to be lacking when it comes to writing articles and papers. The real objectivity comes with the editors' and external reviewers' comments, and this can be hard to take, but it is wise to assume that they are given with goodwill and to try to amend the paper in the light of the comments made. Editors are gatekeepers, selecting the good articles and rejecting those either below the required standard or containing material which is inappropriate for their journal. Papers are normally accepted that are considered to be the following:

- original work
- scientifically sound
- relevant to the readership
- not previously published.

In return the publishers have a duty to handle work sensitively, and within reasonable time-scales. The peer review system used by journals has been justifiably criticised, and it is up to the editor to facilitate unbiased and collaborative working so as to further information sharing to a sustainable standard. Certainly I have found reviewers' comments invaluable, and know from my work as an editor that many very senior academics have appreciated the thought and attention given to improve their work. The firm reject is, of course, the hardest to bear but many a good author has been the recipient of one or more of these, so if your work is rejected either try another outlet or start again. I can say this with feeling! My first attempt at getting published in the nursing press failed miserably, not least perhaps because I was addressing the wrong subject for the readership. I then sought advice from an expert and modified the article for a medical journal. Probably because my supervisor was on the editorial board it was accepted, indeed it was often quoted as a result of its publication, with requests coming from overseas for offprints! Once the glass ceiling is smashed there is a knock-on effect, which means you are kept busy for some time, if that's what you want. Seek the help of known experts; consider being a second author for a first try. One thing is for sure, no journal is going to jeopardise its reputation by publishing poor-quality material, so it is not just a matter of whom you know, although that can help to open doors.

Getting published is exciting – it brings a new dimension to your work and opportunities for interaction with fellow professionals. How you take that dimension forward is up to you, but the possibilities are endless, from developing a certain amount of authority at a local level to developing your own website, to speaking at conferences and contributing to major publications. It is not only your own professional development that is being enhanced but also the development of those around you. However, none of these will bear much fruit if the researcher hides behind long-winded and formal reports and fails to bring them into the practice domain. While I am not suggesting that research findings should be 'dumbed down' in a manner which belittles either the scientific credibility of the work or the intelligence of the potential consumers I am promoting the idea that an approach which will appeal to them should be used, one that relates the research in question to the reader. An example of presentation which comes to mind is that of ballet. Very few balletomanes would watch with pleasure a performance of Swan Lake if the agony of the barre work and the bleeding toes were exposed. However, the mastery and expertise of professional dancers, the hallmark of any fine performance, are easily visible to any observer and so they should be to the research report reader.

Breaking the barriers: User-friendly connections with practice

In the introduction I touched on some of the factors which produce the uncomfortable, indeed negative, effect of research on the population whom the research is supposed to serve. They have, as we have already mentioned, their own pressures and may resent the implication that their input could be improved, or may feel a lack of confidence in considering research in their field. Then, on the inside of the ivory tower there are the academics – striving to bring new learning to health care, pressed to bring in funding, pressed to publish in quality journals to indicate sound peer review, and so on. The ivory, were it transparent, would make it clear to those either side of the wall that neither functions well without the other.

Titchen and Binnie (1993) provided seminal examples of research strategies in practice areas, including action research, and the basis for much of the later work carried out in the nursing development units. Despite these forays into bridging the gulf between practice and research the impact has been minimal in comparison with the effort. Freshwater and Rolfe (2001) and Jarvis (2000) have argued for a practitioner–researcher based approach as a way of managing this dichotomy. This is based on a pragmatic epistemology which values both inductive and deductive knowledge and skills. As a senior nurse seconded full-time to undertake a doctorate Coombs (1999) argues that there needs to be a higher professional commitment to research by practitioners. She makes a case for increased facilitation of research and its application by educationalists and for specific dissemination strategies which are clearly articulated by researchers, and this aspect is taken up in Chapter 6. Coombs's views were sustained by her unusually privileged position at that time, but it is clear that until the organisational barriers to research-based practice are broken the struggle to change the nursing culture from task-based to one of enquiry will continue.

Kitson et al. (1996) argue that deductively tested knowledge given to practitioners ignores the essential elements of inductive learning, thus missing the context and experience which makes sense of facts. This makes a strong argument for nursing research to be within the clinical environment, and while lecturer–practitioner posts, which offer the opportunity to the incumbents of having a foot in both the academic and clinical camp, are becoming more the norm, they are not without their difficulties. These difficulties of either not belonging in either camp or being overstretched by accepting ownership from both require flexible strategies for working which may not appeal to many. Certainly these are not posts which sustain the individual and as such are used, generally, as stepping-stones in career moves. Nursing has not yet achieved a philosophy of practice that sees the production of research as both the work of every practitioner and a viable nursing career pathway in itself that can and should be pursued by a proportion of nurses within the total workforce. As stated earlier, it is frequently seen as something outside of nursing practice and carried out by those divorced from clinical nursing.

For the majority this will relate to using research, but there is a need to increase the number of research active nurses if the nursing knowledge base is expand in relation to the demand for evidenced-based nursing practice.

Despite the number of specialist posts, such as nurse consultant, practice development and lecturer-practitioner posts, where individuals can be identified as playing a part in developing and maintaining a research and development infrastructure and a culture for the use and production of research, there remains a lack of a generally cohesive and clear relationship between academic and other departments and practice areas. Much depends on personalities and opportunism rather than accepted standards.

Accreditation for nursing research in the NHS

We have discussed obliquely throughout this book, and clearly in Chapter 5, some mechanisms and roles which can currently be applied and developed to break through barriers in a move towards a cultural sea change in research awareness. Perhaps one of the most exciting initiatives is one which is currently underway, facilitated by the Royal College of Nursing R&D director. Building on earlier work carried out in conjunction with trust nurse executives (McMahon, Bishop and Shaw, 2000) a small group of experts from across the UK met at the Royal College of Nursing to explore the merits of an accreditation system in NHS trusts in relation to nursing research and development. The group, at the time of writing, are pursuing an inclusive agenda and will work through an iterative process to develop robust standards against which performance can be measured and benchmarked. They consider that nursing cannot advance its contribution to effective health care without research and development, and consider that promoting excellence in R&D in nursing will:

- enable excellence in the delivery of nursing practice and im-prove public health/patient's experiences and outcomes
- improve recruitment and retention
- improve trust performance ratings.

This group accepts that nursing, along with other health dis-ciplines, is committed to a philosophy of evidence-based practice and envisages the roles of research and development as having importance and value. They maintain the long-held view that these activities should be seen as an essential and integral part of nursing activity and that all nurses should therefore develop skills in accessing and using research. It is recognised that research that can underpin nursing practice comes from many disciplines and paradigms. However, the group are firm in their view that nursing is different from other health profession and needs its own unique knowledge base. History has shown that the health research agenda would not further the nursing knowledge base if left to other professional groups and to a generic R&D agenda. Indeed it is acknowledged that there is a current shortfall in nursing research capacity in the UK (Higher Education Funding Council for England, 2001) and that the ratio of nurses currently research active to total nurses in comparison to the ratio of research active doctors to total doctors is very low. This position is seen by many as unacceptable and a view is held that a priority should be placed on increasing both the amount of nursing research and on the number of research active nurses. New postdoctoral scholarships have been set up by several agencies and institutes of higher education to plug some of the gap, but nursing still occupies the rough grassland in a small corner of the research field.

If nursing is to play its rightful role in influencing the quality of health care in the UK a clearer strategy is needed at service level. Although some robust nursing research is available to inform practice there is a shortfall of nursing research available in relation to many core nursing activities. There is a strong view currently being explored more widely that one way to increase the number of research active nurses, the numbers of nurses informing the overall R&D strategy, and the number consciously and explicitly using research as part of practice, is to develop standards and guidelines relating to research and development in clinical practice.

These could be used as part of an accreditation system of trusts, and primary teams. A fundamental aspect of such guidelines would be access to and maintenance of the skills that enable nurses to both access and utilise research-based knowledge in their decision making. At the time of writing the outcome of consultations cannot be gauged, but the activity alone will stimulate fresh thoughts which will undoubtedly have a profound affect on the nursing professions.

The student and the novice researcher is at the threshold of a highly charged and exciting period. The threads of nursing history are drawing together, and the pull of policy versus professional aspirations strengthen the tension. The phrase 'publish and be damned' will, for nursing and the allied professions, change to 'publish and be counted'. Make a difference.

Key points

- The knowledge that nursing has is vital to health care
- Dissemination is the crucial link between research and practice
- New knowledge must be accessible to those who can use it
- Research findings need to be made available at all levels from policy makers to practitioners and users and carers

References

Albert, T. (2000) *Winning the publications game* (2nd edn) Oxford: Radcliffe Medical Press.

Bogdan, R.C. and Bicklen, S.K. (1982) *Qualitative research for education. An introduction to theory and methods.* Boston: MA Allyn and Bacon.

Carr-Hill, R., Dixen, P., Gibbs, I., Griffiths, M., Higgins, M., McCaughan, D. and Wright, K. (1992) *Skill Mix and the effectiveness of nursing care.* York: Centre for Health Economics, University of York.

Coombs, M. (1999) Building bridges between nursing research and practice. In Bishop, V. (ed.) *Working towards a research degree.* London: Emap Publications.

DoH (Department of Health) (1999) *Making a difference. Strengthening the nursing, midwifery and health visiting contribution to health and health care.* London: DoH.

FoNS (Foundation of Nursing Studies) (1996) *The Utilisation of Research in Nursing: A Report of a Phenomenological Study Involving Nurses and Managers.* London: FoNS.

Freshwater, D. (1998) From acorn to oak tree. A Neoplatonic Perspective of Reflection and Caring. *The Australian Journal of Holistic Nursing.* **5**(2): 14–19.

Freshwater, D. and Broughton, R. (2001) Research and Evidence based practice. In Bishop, V. and Scott, I. (eds) *Challenges in Clinical Practice.* Basingstoke: Palgrave – now Palgrave Macmillan.

Freshwater, D. (2002) *Therapeutic Nursing.* London: Sage.

Freshwater, D. and Rolfe, G. (2001) Critical reflexivity: A politically and ethically engaged research method for nursing. *NTResearch*, **6**(1): 526–37.

Froggatt, K., Corner, J. and Bredin, M. (2002) Dissemination and utilisation of an intervention to manage breathlessness: Letting go or letting down? *Nursing Times Research*, **7**(3): 223–31.

Gibran, K. (1965) *A Third Treasury of Khalil Gibran*. New Jersey: Citadel.

Hicks, C. (1994) Of sex and status: a study of the effects of gender and occupation on nurses' evaluations of nursing research. *Journal of Advanced Nursing*, **17**: 1343–9.

Hicks, C. (1995) The shortfall in published research. A study of nurses' research and publication activities. *Journal of Advanced Nursing*, **21**: 594–604.

Higher Education Funding Council for England (2001) *Promoting research in nursing and the allied health professions*. London: HefCE.

Hochschild, A. (1983) *The managed heart*. Berkeley, CA: University of California Press.

James, N. (1993) Division of emotional labour. Disclosure in cancer. In Fineman, S. (ed.) *Emotion in organisations*. London: Sage.

Jarvis, P. (2000) The practitioner–researcher in nursing. *Nurse Education Today*, **20**: 30–5.

Kitson, A., Ahmed, L.B., Harvey, G., Seers, K. and Thompson, D. (1996) From research to practice: one organisational model for promoting research-based practice. *Journal of Advanced Nursing*, **23**: 430–40.

McMahon, A., Bishop, V. and Shaw, T. (2000) *Report of a workshop held at the Royal College of Nursing Annual Nursing Research Conference*. London: RCN.

Martin, C.R., Bowman, G.S., Knight, S. and Thompson, D.R. (1998) Progress with a strategy for developing research in practice. *Nursing Times Research*, **3**(1): 28–34.

Menzies, I.E.P. (1970) *The functioning of social systems as a defence against anxiety*. London: Tavistock Institute.

Nightingale, F. 1980 (1859) *Notes on Nursing*. London: Churchill Livingstone.

NTResearch (1998) Proceedings of the NTResearch Symposium for Evidence-Based Nursing. *NTResearch*, **3**(1): 8–29.

Rafferty, A.M., Traynor, M. and Lewison, G. (2000) Measuring the outputs of nursing R&D: A third working paper. London: Centre for Policy in Nursing Research, London School of Hygiene and Tropical Medicine.

Richardson, A., Jackson, C. and Sykes, W. (1990) *Taking research seriously*. London: HMSO.

Salvage, J. (1998) Evidence based practice; a mixture of motives. *Nursing Times Research*, **3**(6): 406–18.

Scottish Executive (2002) *Choices and Challenges: The strategy for research and development in nursing and midwifery in Scotland*. Edinburgh: www.scotland.gov.uk.

Simpson, M. (1971) Research into nursing problems. In Lord Birkenhead, Williams, E. and McLachlon, G. (eds) *Portfolio for health. Research and Development*. Oxford: Oxford University Press.

Smith, P. (1992) *The emotional labour of nursing*. London: Macmillan – now Palgrave Macmillan.

Tarling, M. (1998) Publish and be damned. In Tarling, M. and Crofts, L. (eds) *The essential researcher's handbook*. London: Balliere Tindall.

Titchen, A. and Binnie, A. (1993) Research partnerships in collaboration: action research in nursing. *Journal of Advanced Nursing*, **18**: 858–65.

11 Looking ahead: The future for nursing research

Veronica Bishop and Dawn Freshwater

> In politics, it matters supremely how we see, think, feel and speak, in other words how we communicate matters. To acknowledge this is the first step towards any kind of action or change of attitude. (Tschudin, 1999:133)

In this chapter we draw on a dialogue between the two editors and discuss the state of nursing today. This involves consideration of the professionalism of nursing; the autonomy of its practitioners and the research programmes needed to support future directions. We identify international and national trends which underpin the current status of nursing research today and seek to promote an agenda for change which is drawn from existing opportunities and planned policy initiatives.

Introduction

It would be too easy in this chapter for two very committed nurses who have strong views on what nursing is and is not to fall into the trap of 'blue sky gazing' and wishful thinking. This is, of course, incongruent with the aims and objectives of this book, nor can we afford to go where others have gone before, and no doubt will again, in trying to define what nursing is. Rather we will leave that debate for other scholars currently engaged in redefining the practice and focus of nursing (see Royal College of Nursing work in progress, 2003). We move on to consider how we may educate nurses in the accumulation of the necessary knowledge to become true professionals with the skills to practice autonomously. Here we might pause and ask, what are the characteristics of a 'professional'? In brief a professional is a person involved in an activity that provides society with a specific service in an institutionalised manner, that has a collective body of knowledge, requires accredited or licensed education and training, and allows that for the individual practitioner to exercise their profession in an autonomous way.

In the first two chapters of this book we considered the context of professional knowledge, with particular focus on nursing research. What are the research approaches most appropriate for the developing nursing profession to underpin and develop further its contribution to its knowledge base? To take forward this debate we discuss the current international status of nursing and then attempted to pinpoint where nursing research appears to have progressed the furthest in relation to our views on where the nursing agenda should be focused. Building on this discussion we then attempt to identify why this may be the case and what the apparent supportive factors were. We then consider how this progress can be built upon by the new generation of professionals. The role of the World Health Organisation (WHO), the International Council of Nurses (ICN) and the Workgroup of European Nurse Researchers (WENR) are briefly but importantly considered in this equation, and the role of the RCN and the Council of Deans in the UK is discussed in the promotion of nursing research. Are the existing mechanisms being used to further the nursing agenda, particularly in terms of research activity and uptake and, if not, what new mechanisms could be put into place?

International trends

An excellent summary of European policies in relation to nursing and nursing research is given by Keighley (2003), who highlights a lack of cohesion in overall health care policy which, of course, has a knock-on effect on nursing, to its detriment. This lack of progress in the largest of all workforces in a vital area of social importance undoubtedly stems not only from overall weakness in central policy making but also from gender issues, a theory particularly well developed by Oakley (for example, 1984), and built upon by Davies (1986) and Salvage (1987). While in many countries the subservience of women is supposed to have become a thing of the past we suggest that much of the albeit slow move to equality in the UK is due to the inclusion of more male nurses in the predominantly female profession.

At the 54th World Health Assembly (WHO) held in March 2001 the member states were urged to strengthen nursing and midwifery through strategies that included closer involvement of these two professions in health care policy, stressing that they had a pivotal role in health care initiatives. It was noted that what was termed significant progress had been made in the development of national nursing and midwifery strategies. It was also noted that while the overall number of training fellowships had increased there was, none the less, a reported shortfall of opportunities compared with the demand. There were, at that time, 35 WHO collaborating centres for nursing and midwifery throughout the world. Their main areas of interest are bedded in capacity building, curriculum development and collaborative research. The need to promote approaches, models and guidelines that are evidence based was stressed but, given the nature and organisation of WHO, which is very medically dominated and dependent on funding from member states for massive programmes of health across disparate continents, it is our view little is likely to emanate from here that is progressive in terms of specific nursing issues.

The International Council of Nurses (ICN) has far more potential, we think, for taking the vision of autonomous practitioners forward and making it a reality. In our view it is limited by the fact that membership is only through the recognised professional body of each member country, in the case of the UK via the Royal College of Nursing. We would like to see the membership to be a little more representative of nurses from the NHS itself and from the academics serving them, rather than only through a trade union, valuable though that is. There is a double-edged sword here, as the UK Royal College, the organisation presumed to be accountable for excellence in UK nursing, is also the largest nursing trade union in the country. In our view this position serves neither aspect well, and a case could well be made that the current situation has a debilitating effect on academic and clinical nurses. Putting, for the moment, that thorny issue aside, it was through the auspices of the ICN that the Workgroup of European Nurse Researchers (WENR) was formed in the 1970s. This organisation has a roving secretariat and holds research conferences biannually in Europe which are generally well attended by delegates from across the globe, particularly from Europe. The aims of WENR are to strengthen the role of nurse researchers in order to promote optimum health care. This objective has recently been supported further by the creation by the ICN of a research network, available through the net (http://www.icn.ch/resnetbul). This network aims to enhance linking and information exchange, with particular focus on advanced nursing knowledge and practice. It is envisaged that it will provide an evolving forum and global resource which identifies trends in nursing and health research and will promote current research, thus strengthening the research agenda globally. While it could not be said that WENR has made a great impact on the society of nursing to date, mainly owing to the costs of travel and time for all member colleagues, it may be, thanks to electronic access, that WENR's time has now arrived. We are excited by this development and will watch (and support where possible) developments. It is certainly an excellent opportunity for nurses with access to the web to contribute to, and benefit from, the research information available. However, it will not provide the opportunity readily for the necessary debate to develop new philosophies which can underpin a united strategy. This in our view is what is missing across the spectrum of organisations and countries, although there are fragments of a strategy which, with good leadership, could be pulled together. It is these that we intend to highlight through our discussion.

UK initiatives

In considering nursing research activity across Europe and judging by the amount of literature published, it appears that with some exceptions we are a little ahead in the UK, but this is not necessarily the case when comparing the UK with the US. We considered the tendency of UK nurses to follow the US trends in education and research, despite having our own far earlier tradition of nursing – or maybe because of it. When talking around this we arrived at the view that while UK nurses do have a tendency to follow the footsteps of American nurses, particularly in grasping new philosophies and theories to guide practice, and while they are not always relevant to care this side of the Atlantic, Americans often seemed to define nursing in a much clearer way through their theories. The lack of tested nursing theories, particularly in the UK, is a major gap. As Abdellah and Levine (1994:230) argue, 'More knowledge is needed on sources of nursing theory, the components of theories, and the development of theories'. Innovations in this area in the UK are predominantly in the area of reflective theories of nursing practice within which the tacit knowledge can be made explicit and extant. Reflective and reflexive theories of nursing practice require further study in order to establish their capacity to develop models of professional practice.

In following the educational lead spearheaded by the US the UK could be criticised for throwing some of the best of nursing out with the bathwater. Certainly the debate since the move of nurse education into diploma or degree status in Project 2000 (see Meerabeau, 1998; Jowett, Walton and Payne, 1994) the supernumerary position of student nurses in clinical areas and the concomitant decrease in clinical experience has raised as many critics as proponents. There are those who passionately believe that nurses should be educated within the principles of higher education, while some consider that this is merely a ploy to raise professional status and pay. This oversimplification of a deeply diverse and complicated set of issues misses the essence of what nursing has to be in order to achieve its potential. Nursing is not about the collection of degrees, NVQs or any other such marks on paper. It is about providing a huge workforce with the scope and opportunity to be educated to think, to interpret, to communicate and to share very particular and at times intimate skills with a given population, be it other professionals, the sick or the vulnerable. The shape of this workforce cannot remain within the traditional framework. Increase in clinical specialisms, changing demographics in workforce potential and the population to be cared for, and the concomitant clinical pressures make this unrealistic. New methods of working have to be tried and tested, and the role of professionals in all health care disciplines questioned.

It was inevitable in our discussion on the expanding (or is it merely changing?) role of the nurse in this country that our thoughts turned to the role of the nurse practitioners in the US, most of whom have a minimum of a degree at Masters level. This trend for higher degrees in some areas of nursing has been consolidated recently by the ICN, who have drawn up a definition of a nurse practitioner/advanced practice nurse in response to the rapid development of the role in some countries. This follows attempts by the UK Royal College of Nursing to have the role of nurse practitioner formally recognised by the Nursing and Midwifery Council. Hot on the heels of these moves is the introduction in Scotland of that country's first clinical doctorate progamme for nurses and midwives. This programme is designed for staff who wish to remain in clinical practice and hope to make a substantive career as nurses or midwife consultants.

Appropriate definition of roles can only benefit employers and staff alike and clarify what have been very muddy waters in the attempts to formalise career structures in clinical areas and to reward expertise and learning. However, setting aside the differences between consultant nurses and advanced practitioners, it remains the case that there are distinctive changes within the health care system concerning divisions of labour and that nurses are not only extending their roles but are taking on the work previously carried out by others – in particular, doctors. Certainly many of the nurse practitioners in the US carry out tasks which would be taken on in the UK by medical housemen or registrars. This is not to say that these tasks should not be undertaken by nurses: they may be a part of the whole programme of care but in our view they need to be undertaken in a holistic way, as part of an entire nursing assessment and not in a piecemeal manner.

Training or education?

We know that any responsible and reasonably intelligent person can be trained to perform specific tasks, but this does not, and should not, imply understanding of the complexities surrounding that task. Nurses are educated today not just to perform tasks and hone practical and communicative skills but also to understand the significance of a multiplicity of issues surrounding these activities. Today's political currency for change in accordance with professional demands is for any concessions to be tied into what is termed modernisation. Here the penalty of past governments' reduction in doctors has landed on the nurses' table and they are to take over many tasks which were previously carried out by doctors. Various legislative changes have already paved the way for these blurring of roles, not least the legislation for reduction in junior doctors' hours (NHSE, 1991) and the more recent policy signal to fracture traditional professional barriers (DoH, 2000). Multiskilling and multidisciplinary work have been sound-bites for some time. This in itself may or may not be damaging to the patient – we come back to the discussion earlier on the difference between a piecemeal approach to care and a progamme of care devised from a holistic, knowledgeable assessment of the individual to be cared for. What is of particular interest when we are considering the essence of nursing is – who will take up the nursing tasks previously carried out by nurses? Were they never very important? Do we hand them over to unqualified staff, or should we increase our student nurse input with shortened training time so that we have more nurses more quickly? The tremendous shortfall of nursing staff across Europe makes it unethical to recruit from other countries – an experiment none the less tried but with limited success in the UK and undoubtedly to the short-term detriment of the mother countries.

The move to an all-graduate profession with extended education and training is strong in the UK and to change that would be a backward step with negative knock-on effects throughout the health care services. This move does not need to exclude non-academic staff from entering nursing but it does mean that the old two-tier system of nursing staff (enrolled nurses and registered nurses) formally re-enters the workforce debate. But, if we are honest, it never really left it. There have always been different grades of education in nursing and, given high demand, limited resources and the given labour market potential, it is unlikely to change. For the reasons we describe above there need be no problem with this as long as staff have the opportunity to develop within their own capacity and wishes. Of particular relevance at this point in our discussions is the emergence of the NHS virtual university. This would appear to have a similar remit to the abandoned NHS Training Authority and can undoubtedly offer much in the way of credible training material which is easily accessible to NHS staff. We voiced concern, however, that it may be making a mockery of the term 'university', which should be synonymous with learning for knowledge's sake as well for fitting one for employment. As a NHS organisation the focus must be on the needs of the Service rather than the educational enlightenment of the individual. It is this short-term deployment of specific knowledge which concerns us. What is changing for the better, in our view, is the recognition that unqualified staff have an important contribution to make to health care, and that NVQs, among other similar shortened forms of specific training, are now more easily available and transferable.

Developing a profession: A purpose of research

While in the main we applaud the developments described above there still remains the tantalising fact that higher education for nurses can be the bullet in the foot! Nursing is described within the Higher Education Funding Council for England as 'an emerging' profession (*NTResearch*, 2003), and for the registered nurse the union with higher education brings about the dilemma of nursing being urged to take on more medically oriented work rather than grasping or being given (or taking) the opportunity to develop nursing approaches. That qualified nursing is key to the health and care of any population is well rehearsed, not least within these chapters, but we still struggle for the freedom to develop our roles as our precious resources are utilised to plaster over the inadequacies of other professionals. This is a point developed further by Hughes (2003:1) when he states:

> Nurses working in Western health care at the start of the twenty-first century find themselves in a period of rapid and sometimes turbulent organisational change. Often it is not clear whether this represents an opportunity for professional advancement or a threat to existent professional norms and working conditions.

In describing a study on 'Time and space on the hospital ward' (Allen, 2003:51) found that the roles and responsibilities in the division of health care labour appeared to be determined in part by the location in time and space, with little attention to organisational descriptions. It is this flexibility which may be our undoing, a point well made by Wilmot (2003:101) when he considers the vulnerability of the imperious or rigid disciplines.

However, Wilmot goes on to stress that while a good case can be made for striving to ensure that some of the existing diversity is preserved, 'in the case of nursing, it is particularly important that its open and flexible approach to health care is not lost in the process of homogenisation'.

We seem to be caught in a web of strong threads which stem from such sources as gender stereotyping, medical dominance, political game playing, resource deprivation and inadequate professional leadership at many levels (Collinson, 2003; Freshwater et al., 2002; Marriner, 1994) and which conspire to keep us in the place where others would have us. If this seems to offer a very negative view of our profession we would suggest that it offers the converse – once the problems are identified the solutions present themselves; it is the unpicking of the knots that takes the time! Never, in our view, has the time been so rich for nursing research. Never has the map been so clearly laid out, albeit warts and all. It is the honesty of colleagues over the years, raising their heads above the parapet that has broken the stones for the path ahead. It is only by providing the evidence of the value of nursing and its effectiveness that we can hope to keep nursing as a profession rather than a group of piecemeal trained (rather than educated) employees. Doctors and, indeed, midwives do not have this dilemma, as their interventions are generally discrete and measurable within the accepted parameters of conventional science. Nursing, in contrast, performs numerous interventions, often simultaneously, and rarely in isolation from other activities. Further difficulties arise for the profession in examining itself and its role in providing optimum health care in the fact that the body of evidence that is being accumulated to support nursing interventions is being developed along the same lines as is investigated for evidence-based medicine. Doing this will just perpetuate the current situation of nursing not having a strong voice in policy and not being counted.

We considered whether or not having a nursing research council would help – a scenario well rehearsed by Rafferty, Bond and Traynor (2000) – and this is an issue which we approach in an oblique way later in the conclusion. It is critical for the profession, in order to meet the criteria of a profession and for greater assurance of knowledgeable care for patients and clients, to work with students on the fundamentals of autonomous practice.

The challenges

Nursing, research, and policy

Despite the fact that many policy decisions directly affect the nursing workforce nurses often perceive themselves to be excluded from the processes of health policy making. These same professionals complain of a gap between policy and practice and indeed policy and research, particularly in terms of the organisation and management of services. *The future of nursing depends not only upon the development of efficient and effective evaluation strategies, but also nurses concerning themselves with policy making at both local and national level.* In this sense practitioners need to develop a commitment to being an epistemic community; that is, a group of professionals who share ideas, values and a dedication to translating ideas into public policy. This could be an extension of clinical supervision and reflective practice with similar processes being used to enable professional practitioners generate policy from their practice.

Barriers to research implementation

Many writers have emphasised the need to close the gap between research and practice in nursing (see, for example, Freshwater and Rolfe, 2001; Burrows and McLeish, 1995; Closs and Cheater, 1994). Simultaneously nursing literature reports the difficulties facing nurses in doing this. The barriers to overcoming the research/practice gap are well documented and are summarised by Freshwater and Broughton (2001). The barriers to the implementation of research findings in practice extend beyond the usual conversations regarding relevance, applicability and transferability of practice knowledge into the culture of nursing itself. In order for nursing to meet the challenge of the twenty-first century it is simply not good enough to plead ignorance of research or passively accept barriers to the implementation of research findings. Nurses have been and will continue to be accountable for their nursing interventions and must be prepared to justify these according to a sound rationale. How and what that rationale is based upon is open to debate and will differ depending upon the particular viewpoint taken, that is, researcher/practitioner – scientist/practitioner. The justification for sound nursing practice may originate in a variety of sources, from professional experience, practice-based research, clinical guidelines and systematic reviews. The important thing is that the rationale, while being developed from a sound basis, is also viewed with an informed scepticism so that everyday nursing practice is left open to a continuous and dynamic exploration. Nurses need to think carefully about whether they should adopt the principles of evidence-based practice to guide their own practice.

Discussion

It seems that the nursing profession is at a very important point in its development and one which requires careful consideration if it is not just to survive but also to grow. We consider this point in time to be of particular significance, perhaps on a par with the nurse Registration Act of 1919, because wrong-footedness in the next few years will see the demise of a noble concept. Central to where nursing is now is consideration of the purpose of nursing in a multidisciplinary professional team. From this question must flow the role of nursing research. If it is not to inform, improve and support that role it is unlikely to be of relevance to the profession. If nursing is to remain a practice-based profession the research must reflect that focus. If it is not to remain a practice-based discipline, what is its focus? The question as to the purpose of the qualified nurse's role in the health care team is not a flippant one. The move of nurse education and training into higher education has raised enormously the potential of 'thinking, knowledgeable doers' but the reverse of this advantage is that student ownership of professional knowledge is diluted, or worse, dispersed by the interests of other disciplines. This confusion or lack of clarity is maintained, indeed strengthened when the newly qualified nurse find that his or her 'profession' is multi-layered and has no clear identity. Nursing is very vulnerable in this respect whereas in other health care disciplines, where there is a single entry gate, there is greater internal coherence; internal coherence links to strong ideas of professional identity and requirements. Nursing, if it hopes to achieve indisputable professional status, needs to consider its criteria for entry and be clear as to its role. It can be seen by the study of the history of nursing, even for just a mere decade, that the nursing profession's flexibility lends itself to the ever-changing winds of demographics and politics. Some may see this flexibility as a strength – it certainly is for those who divide and rule – but it may also be perceived by some as the ongoing barrier to the development of a specific body of workers with a specific body of knowledge. As we write the demand for nurses is such that they are being sought, not without ethical implications, from other countries, and entry criteria to qualification are simplified in a manner which is not compatible with the move of nurse education into higher education. This paradox is at best managed by an unwieldy system of grading or 'levelling'. The pride in becoming a nurse, the feeling of having achieved anything special, may be diminished, and the professional argument for further learning and research mindedness may perhaps seem incongruous. Compounding the difficulties for new nurses, and indeed any who are striving to keep up with the many changes in structures, management and clinical skill requirements, is the lack of role models who are available to staff on a regular basis. By this we mean experienced clinical staff who not only are well qualified but also have organisational memory and sense of context and who can provide formal or informal leadership. The nurse consultant posts may go some way to meet this need, but with so much expected of so few, and over such large areas, the potential of such posts may not be fully realised.

Discussion of role models leads quite naturally to the debate about elitism. The fear of being elitist can be cunningly used by politicians and by individuals to render the playing field below sea level. Nurse researchers are often seen by the main body of nurses as elitist, and the word is not used with affection but rather to undermine. Of course much of this will emanate from the researchers themselves – how available are they, or their works?; have they invented a language which is incomprehensible to the non-researcher? But much also stems from straightforward feelings of resentment by the practitioners. It is an important issue and one which, if not addressed by both the researcher and the practitioner, will hinder the profession as a whole.

Another nettle which must be grasped if the profession is to advance as a nursing entity is the recognition that much of the work around care stems from tacit knowledge. While major funding is mostly available for bio-medical research we must have champions of the issues which are key to nursing as well as pursuing multidisciplinary aspect of care. This is gradually happening, and those researchers who have achieved recognition in this area over long and hard-fought times deserve to be applauded.

Finally in our mapping exercise for our profession we come to the issue of leadership, and in particular leadership in nursing research. The Council of Deans, formed in 1997 from the long-standing Association of Professors and Heads of Departments of Nursing and Directors of Nursing Education Groups, is an important forum which is deeply involved with nursing policy and educational issues, not least through its representation at the Joint Ministerial Review of Education and Research in Primary Care Trusts (*NTResearch*, 2003). Despite its lack of accessibility to the average nurse, in January 2003 it was agreed at the AGM, which was attended by over 70 members, that its role would be widened to include the allied health professionals as from September 2003 to function under a new name, Council O Deans and Heads of UK University Faculties for Nursing and Health Professions. This is an interesting development and only time will tell if it is beneficial to the nursing profession as well as to the host institutions.

While the paucity of visible, senior role models in clinical practice has been touched upon, in academia it could be argued that the plethora of new academic departments serves to confuse. For the newcomer to the academic scene the best option is to search all the university websites and see what appeals in terms of geography and presentation. The main forum for nurse researchers is the excellent annual international Royal College of Nursing research conference, which usually attracts hundreds of delegates from many countries and which offers something for the novice to the more senior researcher. Indeed the RCN must take the credit for much of the activity over the past 25 years that has moved nursing research forward. However, over the past few years we have noted that the most senior academics, and almost none of the senior NHS nurses at board level, attend this venue. This is not a criticism of them but a pointer to the need for united, professional collaboration at that level through some forum. We need a clearer picture of the role of PhDs in clinical practice, apart from the nurse consultant role, and a more empowered body of academics who are supported in their drive to strengthen nursing care in the health services. In our very personal opinion that this is the remit of a Royal College, but not that of a trade union.

These last few paragraphs are encapsulating the discussions of many colleagues over the past years. Many of the points raised in this final chapter may meet opposition, and that is healthy. Considered argument is good between colleagues and should help to move the health care agenda forward on a more thoughtful foundation, with the role of nursing more firmly anchored. The answers lie in the hands of the new professionals, and this is how it should be. It is in our gift to highlight the pitfalls and the potential – it is your prerogative to lead the new way. The potential to do this has been around for a while. Now is the time to take hold of the opportunities, and if this book helps people to do that then we have achieved what we set out to do.

Key points

- The future of nursing as a profession depends on research-based practices.
- Nurses must be politically and strategically aware to maximise the nursing contribution to health services.
- Leadership, to be effective, must be visible.
- Ownership of nursing *by* nurses is the only professional way forward.

References

Abdellah, F.G. and Levine, E. (1994) *Preparing Nursing Research for the 21st Century. Evolution, Methodologies, Challenges.* New York: Springer.

Allen, D. 2003 Time and space on the hospital ward: shaping the scope of nursing practice. In Allen, D. and Hughes, D. (eds) *Nursing and the division of labour in health care.* Basingstoke: Palgrave Macmillan.

Allen, D. and Hughes, D. (2003) Expanded nursing roles: different occupational perspectives. In Allen, D. and Hughes, D. (eds) *Nursing and the division of labour in health care*. Basingstoke: Palgrave Macmillan.

Burrows, D. and McLeish, K. (1995) A model for research based practice. *Journal of Clinical Nursing*, **4**(4): 243–7.

Closs, J. and Cheater, F. (1994) Utilisation of nursing research: Culture, interest and support. *Journal of Advanced Nursing*, **19**(4): 762–73.

Collinson, G. (2003) The primacy of purpose and the leadership of nursing. *NTResearch*, **7**(6): 403–11.

Davies, C. (1995) *Gender and the Professional Predicament in Nursing*. Buckingham: Open University Press.

DoH (Department of Health) 2000. A Health Service of all the talents: Developing the NHS workforce. Consultation document on the review of workforce planning. DoH Online http://www.doh.gov.uk/wfprconsult

Freshwater, D. and Broughton, R. (2001) Research and evidence based practice. In Bishop, V. and Scott, R. (eds) *Challenges in clinical practice*. Basingstoke: Palgrave – now Palgrave Macmillan.

Freshwater, D. and Rolfe, G. (2001) Critical Reflexivity: A politically and ethically engaged research method for nursing. *NTResearch*.

Freshwater, D., Walsh, L. and Storey, L. (2002) Developing leadership through clinical supervision in prison healthcare. *Nursing Management*, Feb.

Hughes, D. (2003) *Nursing and the Division of Labour in Healthcare*. Basingstoke: Palgrave Macmillan.

Jowett, S., Walton, I. and Payne, S. (1994) *Challenges and change in nurse education – a study of the implementation of Project 2000*. Slough: National Federation for Educational Research in England and Wales.

Keighley, T. (2003) Nursing's role in shaping European health policy. In Tadd, W. (ed.) *Ethical and Professional Issues in Nursing: Perspectives from Europe*. Palgrave Macmillan, Basingstoke.

Marriner, A.C. (1994) Theories of Leadership. In Hein, C.E. and Nicholson, M.J. *Contemporary leadership behaviour* (4th edn). Philadelphia: Lippincott Company.

Meerabeau, L. (1998) Project 2000 and the nature of nursing knowledge. In Abbott, P. and Meerabeau, L. (eds) *The Sociology of the Caring Professions* (2nd edn). London: UCL Press.

NHSE (National Health Service Management Executive) (1991) *Junior Doctors: The New Deal*. London: NHSE.

NTResearch (2003) Diary dates from the Council of Deans. *NTResearch*, **8**(3): 228.

Oakley, A. (1984) The importance of being a nurse. *Nursing Times*, **80**(50): 24–7.

Rafferty, A.M., Bond, S. and Traynor, M. (2000) Does nursing, midwifery and health visiting need a research council? *NTResearch*, **5**(5): 325–36.

Royal College of Nursing (2003) *Defining Nursing*. London: Royal College of Nursing.

Salvage, J. (1987) *Nurses, Gender and Sexuality*. London: Heinemann Nursing.

Tschudin, V. (1999) *Nurses matter; reclaiming our professional identity*. Basingstoke: Macmillan – now Palgrave Macmillan.

Wilmot, S. (2003) *Ethics, Power and Policy. The future of nursing in the NHS*. Basingstoke: Palgrave Macmillan.

World Health Organisation (2001) Report by the Secretariat, 30 March. Geneva: World Health Organisation.

Index